MEDICAL CARE
IN THE
UNITED STATES

edited by ERIC F. OATMAN

THE REFERENCE SHELF
Volume 50   Number 1

THE H. W. WILSON COMPANY
New York   1978

THE REFERENCE SHELF

The books in this series contain reprints of articles, excerpts from books, and addresses on current issues and social trends in the United States and other countries. There are six separately bound numbers in each volume, all of which are generally published in the same calendar year. One number is a collection of recent speeches; each of the others is devoted to a single subject and gives background information and discussion from various points of view, concluding with a comprehensive bibliography. Books in the series may be purchased individually or on subscription.

Library of Congress Cataloging in Publication Data
Main entry under title:

Medical care in the United States.

(The Reference shelf ; v. 50, no. 1)
Bibliography: p.
1. Medical care—United States—Addresses, essays, lectures.   2. Medical economics—United States—Addresses, essays, lectures.   I. Oatman, Eric F. II. Series.

RA395.A3M42   362.1'0973   78—4041
ISBN 0—8242—0622—3

PREFACE

Medical care in America has never been more effective—or more expensive. To take one hopeful statistic among many, death rates for men aged fifty-five to sixty-four dropped 12 percent in the period between 1969 and 1975. But during those six years, overall spending on medical care jumped about 85 percent.

The nation's bill for medical care continues to skyrocket. In 1975, it averaged out to $564 for each man, woman, and child in the United States. By 1980 that figure is expected to nearly double—to $1,038. Moreover, residents of inner-cities and of rural areas as often as not find that high-quality medical care is just not available to them at any price close to the average. Doctors, having settled elsewhere, are out of reach.

Many experts, in and out of government, feel that the cost of medical care is dangerously high—affordable by too few. Today, the average American worker puts in one month's work each year to pay for medical care. The federal government, for its part, spends 12 cents of every taxpayer dollar to support health-care programs (including Medicare and Medicaid), to develop health resources through research, personnel training, and facility construction, and to prevent and control health problems.

And if the cost of medical care should double? What then? To economists, the answer is obvious. Individuals would have less money left over for other necessities such as housing, food, clothing, and education. And the government would have less to spend on the other services it provides: everything from highways to defense to flood relief and aid to education. Worse, perhaps, millions of Americans who can afford medical care today could be priced out of the market.

In the light of this scenario, it seems a paradox that relatively so few Americans concern themselves with the problems of the nation's unique system of medical care. Yet, for reasons this volume will attempt to clarify, most Americans are insulated from those problems. Most Americans have ready access to medical care. Furthermore, the impact of potentially devastating medical bills is often absorbed by a "third-party payer"—a private (or public, in the case of the aged and the indigent) insurer. Sombody else is paying the bill.

Or so it seems. Dr. Barry Commoner, the ecologist, reminds us that there is no such thing as a free lunch. Certainly this principle holds true in medical care. The fact is that whether they pay directly or through higher insurance premiums and higher taxes, individual Americans pay for their own medical care—and for the medical care of others.

Medical-care costs and efforts to control them will be a focal point of this volume. But other issues central to medical care in America demand equally close scrutiny.

The material in this volume has been arranged in two main parts. Part One, "The Issues," introduces the major issues of medical care in America. Section I explores the question of quality: How good is medical care in America? The selections in Section II sketch the anatomy of medical-care costs. Section III explains how methods of financing the system can create problems of their own. Section IV addresses itself to the plight of those who live in areas that are short of medical resources; it closes with a discussion of the concept that medical care is a citizen's right—like the right of free speech or free assembly—to be protected and advanced by the federal government.

Part Two, "The Search for Answers," looks at the responses proposed to questions raised in Part One. Section V considers various proposals for a system of national health insurance. Section VI reviews the contributions of health maintenance organizations (HMOs). Finally, in Section VII, two articles assess the relevance to the United States of Britain's National Health Service and Sweden's highly praised system of medical care.

A word of caution. This volume's title speaks of medical care, not health care. Medical care involves the restoration of health to individuals who are sick; health care is a more ambitious undertaking, concerned with keeping the community healthy by preventing sickness as well as curing it. The distinction has been observed by the compiler of this volume. In a few places, however, authors of some of the material inadvertently blur the distinction, using the terms *medical care* and *health care* interchangeably.

The compiler wishes to thank those authors and publishers who were kind enough to let their materials be reprinted in this book. He is especially indebted to his wife, Jane, and to his daughter, Alison, for their patience during the preparation of the manuscript.

ERIC F. OATMAN

January 1978

CONTENTS

PREFACE 3

PART ONE: THE ISSUES
I. THE QUESTION OF QUALITY

Editor's Introduction 11
Robert B. Greifinger and Victor William Sidel. Three
    Centuries of Medical Care .... Environment 12
Unfit Doctors .... New York Times 26
Patrick Young. Your Doctor Is Cramming ....
.... National Observer 30
How Nurses Rate Hospital Care .... Time 34

II. THE QUESTION OF COSTS

Editor's Introduction 37
Matt Clark and others. Health-Cost Crisis .. Newsweek 38
Christine E. Bishop. Paying the Doctor ....
.... Current History 44
Maurice Fox. Why People Are Mad at Doctors ......
.... Newsweek 46
James L. Goddard. Costly Drugs and Supplies ....
.... Scientific American 49
Abigail Trafford Brett. The Cost of Technology ......
.... U.S. News & World Report 59

III. THE QUESTION OF PAYMENT

Editor's Introduction 67
Martin Feldstein. Hospital Costs and Insurance ......
.... Public Interest 68

Dorothy P. Rice. Public and Private Financing ......
.... Current History   75
John P. Allegrante. Uninsured in America ....
.... New York Times   77
Leda R. Judd. Medicaid Programs .... Current History   79
David C. Berliner. Medicaid Abuse ....
.... Washington Post   81
Robert W. Merry. Medicaid Retrenchment ....
.... National Observer   84
Leda R. Judd. Medicare .... Current History   86
Lawrence Mosher. The "Rich" Medicare Docs ......
.... National Observer   87

IV.   THE QUESTION OF AVAILABILITY

Editor's Introduction   90
Mary W. Herman. Health Care and the Patient's Needs
.... Current History   91
John B. Dunne. Why Rural Doctors Are Missing ....
.... Blair & Ketchum's Country Journal   103
Paul Starr. Too Many Doctors? ....
.... Working Papers for a New Society   114
Benjamin B. Page. The Right to Health Care ....
.... Current History   124

PART TWO: THE SEARCH FOR ANSWERS

V.   NATIONAL HEALTH INSURANCE

Editor's Introduction   133
Leda R. Judd. Federal Involvement in Health Care
     After 1945 .... Current History   135
Charles C. Edwards. Needed: A National Authority ..
.... Washington Post   144
Richard J. Margolis. The Dream Whose Time Has
     Come? .... New York Times Magazine   148
Martin Feldstein. Major-Risk Insurance ....
.... Public Insterest   158

Sheila McGough. AMA President Discusses Health-Care
  Costs .... National Observer 165

VI.   HEALTH MAINTENANCE ORGANIZATIONS

Editor's Introduction 170
Lee Smith. Kaiser and the "Desert Doctors": A Way to
  Cut Medical Bills .... Dun's Review 171
Containing the Cost of Employee Health Plans—With
  Health Maintenance Organizations ....
  ....., ... Business Week 173
Alan Reynolds. Less May Be Enough ....
  .... National Review 181

VII.   MODELS FROM ABROAD

Editor's Introduction 184
Joseph G. Simanis. The British National Health Service
  .... Current History 185
Joseph L. Andrews Jr. Medical Care in Sweden ......
  .... JAMA
  (Journal of the American Medical Association) 191

BIBLIOGRAPHY 204

PART ONE: THE ISSUES

I. THE QUESTION OF QUALITY

EDITOR'S INTRODUCTION

How good is medical care in America? To many, this is *the* issue, the only question in the medical-care debate that needs answering. Why worry about costs and the availability of doctors, they wonder, if the product being sold—curative medicine—is shoddy? Why debate the cost of a system that does not deliver the cures it promises? Better to scrap the system, they say, and start over.

Fortunately, for the most part the quality of medicine practiced in the United States is very high. US doctors are as well trained as any in the world, and they work with the best equipment. This permits them to be as accurate and thorough as current knowledge will allow. Advances in pharmacology, surgery, and therapeutic techniques have given US doctors a potent arsenal against disease.

The opening article in this section, taken from *Environment*, gives an overview of three centuries of medical care in America and points up the fact that the present medical system is a product of its own history and values. The struggle for health continues—and sometimes falters. Our medical care system contains embarrassing lapses and deficiencies, side by side with some miraculous successes. The authors maintain that past and present social forces shaping the health-care system must be taken into account if any efforts to produce change are to be effective.

On the debit side are the numbers of doctors unfit to practice. The second selection, from the New York *Times*, estimates their number at sixteen thousand. However, there are encouraging signs that the medical profession has taken steps to purge its ranks of the unfit. One step is periodic

examinations for recertification of family doctors, the subject of the third article, "Your Doctor Is Cramming," by
Patrick Young, a staff correspondent for the *National Observer*.

The section concludes with an article from *Time* entitled "How Nurses Rate Hospital Care," based on a survey
of ten thousand nurses. Their answers to the question add
up to what the article describes as "a disturbing diagnosis."

THREE CENTURIES OF MEDICAL CARE [1]

During the seventeenth century, most of the immigrants
to North America [came] . . . with the purpose of establishing a "City of God on Earth." Medical care at that time had
no prospects of cure as we know it but rather a special kind
of preventive approach. It was believed that . . . by leading a
life compliant with fundamental law, replete with produc-
tive works for one's family and community, a person could
have health, satisfaction, and maintenance of his covenant
with God. There were, of course, many remedies for relief
of pain and of some other symptoms of illness, but there
were no major attempts to interfere with what was seen as
God's will.

The early settlers and their several succeeding genera-
tions relied on the post-Renaissance understanding of the
world as a combination of four substances—fire, air, water,
and earth—and on a view of human physiology as a har-
mony of four humours—black bile (melancholy), green bile
(what we call bile), white bile (mucus), and sanguis (blood).
American native medical care was more complex, not only
in its remedies but also in its methods of controlling what
were seen as positive and negative forces in nature and,
thereby, in the body. Both cultures, however, accepted their

[1] From article entitled "American Medicine," by Robert B. Greifinger and
Victor William Sidel. *Environment*. 18:6–18. My. '76. Reprinted by permission of
Scientists' Institute for Public Information. Copyright © 1976 Scientists' Institute
for Public Information. Greifinger is chief resident in social medicine at Monte-
fiore Hospital and Medical Center in New York City; Sidel is chairman, department of social medicine at Albert Einstein College of Medicine in the Bronx, New
York.

leaders as having spiritual powers for healing, and, in fact, there was little separation of roles in social, religious, and medical hierarchies. . . .

Nevertheless, a number of medical developments were imported from the Old World. As early as 1690, Cotton Mather attempted to have smallpox inoculation (immunization through the use of actual smallpox virus rather than with cowpox virus, as is done today) mandated by law in Massachusetts. This early public health measure was surrounded by tremendous controversy—again, mainly because it was seen as an interference with God's will; it was defeated, which was probably just as well since, by modern standards, the method was unpredictable and dangerous.

Old Beliefs Questioned

By the time of the Great Awakening in the colonies, around 1740, there had been several cultural changes which allowed the development of active intervention in health matters. The view of nature was changing to a more positive one, in line with the view that "all men are created equal," have natural rights, and can realize their potential through assertion and individual achievement. People began to contract with each other for services, thereby accepting the notion that another person could aid an individual's achievement with a specialized service. Folk medicine and self-care were also extremely important. By the late eighteenth century, "patent" medicines, which could be widely publicized through the new technology of printing, were sold on a mass scale in the colonies as well as in England. Manuals for home use, including the Reverend John Wesley's *Primitive Physic*, which went through some thirty editions in England and in America, had wide public appeal.

These Old World patterns underwent major modifications when transplanted to the New World. . . . Most doctors were trained by apprenticeship and practiced general forms of medicine. The small, isolated settlements on the frontier could not support fully trained doctors, and advice on health care came from itinerant peddlers of nostrums, remedies, and balsams of life. Women as well as men could play an important role as healers and had a special role in health care as midwives, since men were usually prohibited from the practice of obstetrics.

In the great seaboard cities, physicians trained in European universities began to challenge the prevalent folk medicine and the doctors who were locally trained by apprenticeship. These European doctors came in increasing numbers to develop an academic, intellectual style of medical care. A medical school on this model was started at the University of Pennsylvania in Philadelphia in 1765, and others followed in New York (1768), Boston (1782), and New Haven (1813). The great American physicians of the time became well-respected leaders, and, in fact, many were representatives in the Continental Congresses and were signers of the Declaration of Independence. Almost the only model available for medical care as the United States of America came into being was entrepreneurial fee-for-service medical care, and little thought was given to medical services provided by local or federal government. Neither public health nor medical care is mentioned in the Constitution, either as powers of the federal government or as powers reserved to the states or to the people. . . .

The nineteenth century brought hospitals, medical schools, and attempts at public health measures. Although by the late eighteenth century in England, hospitals were divided into those for curables and those for the hopeless, hospitals in the United States were largely built for the incurables—for the most part, for poor incurables. People healed or died at home and, in fact, were by all accounts much safer there than in the hospitals, where infectious diseases ran rampant and killed many patients. Nonetheless, hospitals in Philadelphia, New York, and Boston became teaching hospitals and established the tradition of training physicians, surgeons, and nurses within the confines of an institution, outside the medical office and the home. The European-trained professors lectured at length on the medical developments of the time. In the United States, a large part of the hospital's role in curative medicine did not arise until the late nineteenth century, following the development of anesthesia, improved surgical techniques, and a better understanding of human physiology. The general acceptance of the idea that some diseases are caused by microbes and of the value of antisepsis came quite late in the United States, after 1890, forty years after such ideas had been introduced in Europe. . . .

During the period before the Civil War, populism found its medical expression through the widespread practice of lay healing. Lay practitioners preferred treatment with herbs, diet, and human warmth to the more dangerous—and, at that time, not necessarily more effective—ministrations of trained doctors. Women continued to play a significant part in health care as lay practitioners. But by 1830, thirteen state governments—significantly, not the federal government—had passed medical licensing laws outlawing "irregular" practice and establishing trained doctors as the only legal healers. The battle raged in one form or another until the end of the century, when a combination of state and national medical societies, with large funding from foundations, finally drove out much "irregular" practice and with it much of the role of women in medicine.

In the developing cities of the Midwest, small medical colleges appeared, often with little or no equipment or affiliation with hospitals. Physicians were used not only for medical services but also for advice on education, sanitation, and control of infectious disease. They came to be viewed as experts in both prevention and treatment, and, although there came to be some separation of these functions in the largest cities, most doctors did both. Almost all medical practice involved a fee or a payment in kind, such as food or clothing, for the services rendered. But many of the public preventive services were performed solely for the public good; this helped to establish a tradition of charitable medical service in the United States which was prevalent among physicians until the onset of Medicaid legislation 150 years later. As early as 1818 in Germany and 1861 in Russia, physicians were hired by governments to deliver personal medical services and were considered civil servants. Over the next century and a half, this concept spread throughout Europe, but it has never taken root in the United States.

Urban Industrial Diseases

With the Industrial Revolution of the mid-nineteenth century, great numbers of factories appeared, spawning large groups of what we now call the working poor. Mass migrations of Europeans, especially from Ireland during the early nineteenth century, filled the demand for labor in the new factories. Unable to live off their land and often poorly educated, the immigrants clustered in shoddy, congested urban housing. The resulting malnutrition and crowding made these unskilled laborers prime candidates for the diseases of poverty, and infectious diseases were able to spread easily, rapidly, and widely.

Tuberculosis, rickets, and scurvy were endemic among the poor. On the other hand, epidemics of typhus, typhoid fever, yellow fever, smallpox, cholera, and syphilis affected the rich and poor alike. All these diseases were devastating and aroused much public concern. . . . By the mid-nineteenth century, it was recognized that epidemic diseases were promoted by social conditions, especially poverty and crowding, but that the wealthy were not immune to them. These "egalitarian" diseases stimulated interest in disease control; it was recognized that prevention was possible through isolation (quarantine) and sanitation and not only through the ministrations of physicians and surgeons. Thus, the public health movement in the United States began as a reaction to the effects of poverty and has continued, in the areas of sanitation, water supply, and control of communicable diseases, quite apart from personal health services.

Throughout the century preceding the Industrial Revolution in America, European nations had taken a much greater interest in public health measures, resulting in early efforts to control communicable disease and even to provide minimum income through social legislation and government action. . . . Americans, having little sense of reliance on a central government, allowed matters of public welfare to languish until poverty and crowding forced the issue.

Another factor in the mid-nineteenth century which had an impact on the nature of both public and personal medical services was the beginning of registration of causes of death in New York and Massachusetts. The practice of public recording of such statistics was a new one at that time in the United States, although it had been done in Europe and Great Britain for several centuries. . . .

Disease Causes Questioned

Before the Civil War, there were great controversies about the causes of various diseases; these revolved mostly around the miasmic theory, which attributed epidemics to poisonous atmospheric or other environmental conditions, and the specific contagion theory, which postulated specific identifiable causes for each disease. In England and, later, in Germany and France, the two theories were merged, with the understanding that infectious disease arose from a combination of environmental factors and specific contagious factors. The remarkable work of Louis Pasteur and Robert Koch in the identification of specific microbial agents capable of causing disease was interpreted in divergent ways on either side of the Atlantic. The theory prevalent in Europe stressed the interplay of many factors, while the specific agent theory prevailed in the United States. This simplistic acceptance of a single, specific cause for each disease was to prevail until well into the twentieth century in the United States and had considerable impact on the manner in which medical care developed here.

The issue of states' rights was strong in the early nineteenth century, and state and local governments, with the specific agent theories as their major guide, began to feel a responsibility for controlling the spread of bacteria, parasites, and other microorganisms; they felt far less obligation, however, to modify the social conditions which promoted this spread of disease. The states assumed responsibility for treatment of mental disease and tuberculosis, and large public hospitals were built by the cities and the states. Public water supplies and sewage control were taken out of the realm of medical care and began to be managed by engineers. Although the boards of health which were developing in the cities during the pre–Civil War era had an interest in these issues, it was not until after the war that they were given the legal mandate to keep public water supplies clean, to monitor food for contamination, and to quarantine victims of infectious diseases. It was not until thirty years later that health standards were legally required for milk and other foodstuffs. A national board of health was started in 1875, but it was disbanded in 1882 because public health was not considered a province of the federal government.

Physicians and surgeons, who had long commanded respect and power in American society, were faced with a dilemma. Since remarkable changes in health were now available by means of environmental control, would doctors become part of the public-health-care establishment, or would they try to maintain their role outside government? The growing use of anesthetics such as nitrous oxide and chloroform, along with a better understanding of human pathology, brought the opportunity to develop medical services which could be effectively performed on a one-to-one basis. Hospitals, already controlled by physicians, were ideal for both the teaching and the practice of medicine. As a result, the great majority of physicians and surgeons chose to remain outside government and in one-to-one practice.

As in politics, education, and industry, issues of power and control of resources became significant in the post–Civil War development of medical care. During the late nineteenth century, as many as 400 medical schools were founded in the United States; most lasted only a short time, but at least 147 medical schools were operating near the end of the century. These were privately owned institutions, and, lacking standardized graduation requirements, they produced physicians and surgeons who had inconsistent and often inadequate education. Some medical students were trained in European-style schools which offered a combination of humanitarianism and utilization of the knowledge emanating from the major universities regarding the nature and treatment of disease. Others were trained in schools which, by any standards, could only produce charlatans. Local medical societies were organized during the nineteenth century, and in 1847 the American Medical Association (AMA) was formed. It remained until the turn of the century a rather loosely structured organization, mainly concerned with the continuing education of its members.

Rise of the AMA

The twentieth century is the era that will be identified with the explosion of science and technology in medicine and with the concomitant use of power in medical schools and research institutes. The forerunner of the twentieth century pattern was the Johns Hopkins Medical School, formed during the 1890s as an attempt to combine the most advanced knowledge of European universities with skills developed in the United States.

At that time, the teaching faculties of Johns Hopkins and other leading medical schools rose in power within the AMA. In 1901, there was a major reorganization of the AMA; councils were developed, including one on medical education. During the first decade of the century, as the AMA was developing a strong leadership and a large following, it began to take positions on social issues. By 1910, the AMA was concerned with the issue of financing national health insurance, and in a well-publicized statement it indicated that the medical profession ". . . has the responsibility to society . . . and must change for its betterment." In 1916, its committee on social insurance recommended a system of national health insurance. Over a period of twenty years, the AMA had become outspoken on the subject of coordination and equitable distribution of medical services within society. Thus, at a time when power groups such as labor unions were being organized to promote the desires and rights of various segments of the populace, the AMA became the voice of the physician in American society.

At the same time, a radical change in the nature of medical education in the United States was taking place. The Carnegie Commission had authorized Abraham Flexner, a nonphysician, to evaluate medical education throughout the country. In 1910, the Flexner Report disclosed many of the inadequacies in medical education and, within a few years, brought about the closing of many of the "borderline" medical schools. The public was responsive to the report's suggestions that commercialism, incompetence, and avarice should be removed from the practice of medicine and that America should create a new breed of physicians. This advice, however, also had other consequences—the concentration of medical education in the laboratory and hospital rather than in the home and the doctor's office and the concentration of control of medical education by the AMA and other professional organizations.

Science had provided a new vocabulary for the university, and the use of anesthetics had given both credibility and renewed power to practitioners of healing arts. Within a short period of time, surgery became known as a field of curative medicine. These insights, combined with an understanding, in later decades, of specific methods of treatment such as insulin, antibiotics, cortisone, and tranquilizers allowed the development of a power base of persons who could perform services seen as efficacious.

The emphasis on the utilization of scientific theory in medical care, especially in a society wedded to the "single agent theory" of the genesis of illness, developed into a focus on disease and symptoms rather than on therapy, prevention of disability, and caring for the "whole person." The old-fashioned family doctor had viewed patients in relation to their families and communities and had apparently been able to help people cope with problems of personal life, family, and society; the vigor with which American medicine adopted science left many of these qualities in the lurch. Science allowed the physician to deal with tissues and organs, which were much easier to comprehend than were the dynamics of human relationships, being propounded by Sigmund Freud and Carl Jung, or the complexities of disease prevention. Many physicians made efforts to integrate the various roles; however, the main thrust within society was toward academic science.

Public Medical Services

There were other changes in American society which had an impact on the nature of modern medical services. Until the turn of the century, medical care had been relatively inexpensive and accessible, even to the poor. But in the early twentieth century, medical care became more complex, expensive, and limited. At the same time, the urban poor grew in numbers as a result of immigration from Europe and migration from rural areas; the demand for health services for the poor increased. Academic medicine had a use for such people in its teaching and research activities, and in fact the poor in many cases received advanced, specialized medical care on the basis that charity cases were acceptable to physicians as a contribution to medical education.

In addition to the development of publicly supported general hospitals, local governments for the first time became involved in the delivery of specialized personal health services outside the hospital. During the first decade of the twentieth century, New York and, later, other large cities allowed their boards of health to take a special interest in maternal and child health care at the public expense. Efforts were organized around requirements for clean milk and the development of other nutritional programs for children, especially within public schools. . . . School systems around the country were increasingly required to provide medical services for children who were not otherwise receiving them, including children with remediable deficiencies such as poor vision and hearing. Thus began a new era of medical intervention in public institutions, which later developed in some instances into attempts to provide comprehensive care.

Physicians did not escape the profound changes in attitude which followed World War I. The shift in US public opinion toward isolationism, protectionism, and various forms of escapism was reflected within organized medicine. In the early 1920s, the AMA was taken over by a group of physicians very different from those who had espoused national health insurance earlier in the century, and the organization began to function as a much more clearly defined special interest group, leaders of which took control over most community hospitals.

The AMA effectively restricted physician training in the United States by setting limits to the numbers of physicians delivering health services, based on allegedly desirable goals. These quotas had no discernible relationship to health-care needs and instead seemed designed to prevent expansion in the number of physicians. The AMA during this period also began to oppose any effective system of health insurance—with its attendant controls over utilization of services and fees—a stand which has continued to this day.

With the onset of the Depression and the demand for social insurance as differentiated from insurance against specific risks, the United States did not move in the direction which many European countries had taken, that of providing free medical care or reimbursement for its cost. It attempted instead to provide more general social security benefits, unemployment income, federally funded job opportunities, and, to a certain extent, welfare, or "charity," benefits to those with special needs.

What was of great importance to medical care in the Social Security legislation of the 1930s was the shift from local control of health and welfare issues to more centralized control. The cost of caring for children, the elderly, and, subsequently, the poor became the province of the state and federal governments. The ideas of workmen's compensation, pensions, unemployment insurance, and certain kinds of medical services came to be perceived by the people as part of their collective responsibility nationwide. A national health survey was first performed in 1935. A cooperative effort was seen as necessary for recovery from the effects of the Depression and, later, for national defense during the rapid rise of the Nazi power in Europe. The seeds were being sown for the use of health insurance and health services as part of a process of more just distribution of society's resources. . . .

Medical Care Today

. . . Medical care is now a huge part of the American economy, second only to the construction industry in its size and its portion of the Gross National Product, of which it now comprises 8 percent. Five million people are employed in the delivery or support of medical services.

Currently, the most visible and most expensive component of medical care in the United States is hospital care, which is largely based on advanced technology: For example, 780 coronary-care units are available for intensive monitoring of the therapy of moribund cardiac patients; computerized transaxial tomography, a sophisticated, hugely expensive type of X-ray, is available for the purpose of diagnosis without surgery or dangerous drugs; and vital organs can be transplanted from one living person to another. Measures available to the physician include drugs ranging from antibiotics for the treatment of infection to major tranquilizers for mental illness to synthetic hormones. In short, since the beginning of the Industrial Revolution, there has been a tremendous increase in the mass of knowledge (science) and in the development of new products and methods (technology). These changes have resulted in the most expensive medical tradition—and, with the possible exception of Sweden, the most advanced medical technology —in the world.

Despite these remarkable technological achievements— or perhaps because of them—there are problems. Medical technology is centered in the hospital, and thus the major medical services are in hospitals, away from homes and workplaces. There is a concentration on disease rather than on health, which tends to separate medical care from concern for the patient and his family. The power of the technology itself can lead to problems such as adverse drug reactions and injury from equipment or procedures and to ethical dilemmas such as indefinite prolongation of the process of dying. Most physicians in the United States practice specialty medicine, as contrasted with general medicine, a pattern different from every other country in the world. Often, there are varying standards of care for people in different classes or regions. The cost of medical care is high and is increasing; annual per capita cost for medical care now averages $547. The fee-for-service type of practice may lead to much unnecessary surgery and other treatments, with their attendant risks and expense, and quality control is very difficult.

In spite of its technological superiority, the United States lags behind other Western industrialized countries in major health indices. The rate of infant mortality, which is only partly influenced by medical care, has not fallen as rapidly in the United States as it has in other industrialized countries: The US rate of approximately 17 deaths in the first year of life per 1,000 live births now ranks far below Sweden (10 per 1,000) and the Netherlands (11 per 1,000), and the US rate for nonwhite infants is still approximately 30 deaths per 1,000 live births. Concomitantly, . . . life expectancy at birth (a peculiar statistic which is more a reflection of how many of the young and middle-aged die than of how long the elderly live) in the United States has risen dramatically: Philadelphians born in the 1780s could expect to live to age 25; a century ago, Americans had a life expectancy of 41; today, the life expectancy at birth in the United States is 67 for males and 75 for females. Yet Sweden, for example, reports a life expectancy at birth of 72 years for males and 77 years for females.

Context for Change

... Given the history of the United States and the state of its current society, it is not surprising that we have a medical care system which is highly technical, disease-oriented rather than health-oriented, largely fragmented and uncoordinated, and which uses methods of organization which often seem to be based on private gain rather than on the most effective or efficient attainment of the public good.

Since the present medical care system is a product of its own history and values, it is within this context that we must search for ways to change it. Although other countries have in some ways produced systems which are better organized, more efficient, and more effective than ours, these, too, are products of the special circumstances which molded them and cannot be transplanted into alien soil without danger of withering. ...

If the present patterns of medical care are followed, there will be increasing emphasis on technological medicine, growing concentration of resources in hospitals, rapidly escalating costs, but little or no increase in attention to preventive medicine and primary care. Improvements in medical technology and hospital care have advantages for those relatively few individuals who need highly specialized techniques such as organ transplants, cardiac surgery, and sophisticated diagnostics; the problem is that there is a limit to the portion of the Gross National Product which can be allocated to health care. As more resources go into expensive, technologically oriented services, less will remain for *prevention* of both the common diseases and of those diseases which require expensive treatment. Society can no longer avoid questions such as whether funds should be spent on treating a small group of people for a problem which, for the same amount of money, might have been entirely prevented in a much larger group of people. ...

[But] those who would effect change must [first] analyze the past and present social forces which shape the health-care system. Without such analysis, efforts to produce change are likely to be, at best, futile and, at worst, dangerous to our health.

UNFIT DOCTORS [2]

At least 5 percent of the nation's 320,000 doctors are considered by medical authorities to be unfit to practice and may account for tens of thousands of needless injuries and deaths each year. A large proportion of the deaths are the result of unnecessary or incompetently performed operations and faulty drug prescriptions.

Though such conditions have existed for many years, recent studies by professional groups indicate that they are now more widespread than most medical authorities had suspected. Perhaps the greatest obstacle to improving the situation, many experts say, is the traditional reluctance of physicians to criticize and discipline their errant colleagues.

These are the principal findings in a series of New York *Times* stories, written by Boyce Rensberger and Jane E. Brody, exploring the extent and nature of incompetent medical care. What follows is a digest of the stories.

Scope of the Problem

While most of the country's doctors are thought to be relatively competent and conscientious, the Federation of State Medical Boards estimates that at least sixteen thousand definitely are not. They include some who are mentally ill or addicted to drugs as well as others who are simply ignorant of modern medical knowledge or careless in their use of it. Many medical authorities say these doctors, who treat an estimated total of 7.5 million patients a year, should have their licenses revoked, be required to undergo further training or practice only under close supervision.

Doctors and medical judgments cannot always be evaluated directly because, for example, many doctors practice

[2] Article entitled "U.S. Doctors: About 5 Percent Are Unfit." New York *Times*. sec IV, p 11. F. 1, '76. © 1976 by The New York Times Company. Reprinted by permission.

alone and their records cannot be examined, and because diagnoses and therapies must be based on highly subjective evaluations of symptoms and other factors in the patient. Most critics of medical incompetence contend that many avoidable injuries and deaths probably occur in these inaccessible areas.

Studies of the adequacy of medical care reveal a great unevenness from one region to another, from one hospital to another within a region and from doctor to doctor within a single hospital. The studies raise such questions as these:

Why should people be five to ten times as likely to die during a given operation in one hospital than they are in another? Why should the people in one region of a state be three or four times as likely to undergo the most common surgical procedures as people in another similar region of the same state? Such variations, in the opinion of many medical leaders, expose millions of patients to unnecessary risks.

Surgery

At least 250,000 of the approximately 18 million Americans who underwent surgery . . . [in 1975] died during or shortly after their operations, according to the National Center for Health Statistics. Many of these patients were critically ill before the surgery and most probably would have died had they not had an operation. For others, however, it was the operation itself that ended their lives.

The risks of surgery include such postoperative complications as pneumonia, blood clots, shock, infection and hemorrhage, and those associated with anesthesia. General anesthesia—being put to sleep—is considered especially hazardous, since the potent drugs used can interfere with the functions of the respiratory system, the heart and blood vessels, the brain and the kidneys.

A two-year study by the surgical profession of 1,493 patients who suffered complications found that almost half the 1,451 nonfatal complications and a third of the deaths that resulted were preventable. The study, which examined data about patients treated at ninety-five hospitals in seven states, showed that 78 percent of the preventable complications were due to surgeons' errors, with one half resulting from faulty surgical techniques.

The *Times* series cited the following as one example of error:

A man entered a leading New York hospital for the replacement of a heart valve that had been damaged by rheumatic fever. When he was taken off the heart-lung machine after his operation, his circulation failed and he died in minutes. An autopsy disclosed that the surgeon had put the artificial valve in backward, preventing blood from flowing through the heart.

According to findings of a congressional subcommittee, at least 11,900 surgery-related deaths in the United States . . . [in 1975] were entirely avoidable because the surgery was not necessary.

Studies by researchers at such medical centers as Stanford, Cornell and Harvard have indicated that about one in five elective operations—which constitute approximately 80 percent of all surgery performed in the United States—is unneeded.

For some procedures, such as hysterectomies and tonsillectomies, the studies found that as many as one third to two thirds of the operations done may simply not be necessary. Rather, experts who have reviewed the data maintain, these questionable operations are performed because the doctor exercises poor judgment, because the patient insists on or expects surgery or because the doctor wants to protect himself from a possible lawsuit.

Drug Prescriptions

Every year perhaps thirty thousand Americans accept the drugs their doctors prescribe for them and die as a direct result. Perhaps ten times as many patients suffer life-threatening and sometimes permanent side effects, such as kidney failure, mental depression, internal bleeding and loss of hearing or vision.

These figures are projected nationally from local studies and therefore may not be statistically accurate, but they are among the more conservative to be found in studies of the prescription drug problem by the medical profession.

Although patients in the vast majority of cases are helped by the drugs prescribed by them, Dr. John C. Ballin, director of the American Medical Association's Department of Drugs, says: "The literature abounds with references to the prescription of the wrong drug or dose, to unforeseen drug reactions, or simply to the administration of a drug when none is indicated."

Part of the drug reaction problem can be traced to the bewildering variety of drugs available to doctors. About 1,200 different drugs are on the market, many more than any doctor can possibly know well. No drug is completely safe, all have potential side effects, each is intended for a specific use. Yet any licensed doctor is free to use any drug in any way he cares to, regardless of how well or how long ago he has been trained or how diligently or poorly he keeps his knowledge up to date.

Policing the Profession

State licensing agencies over the last thirteen years have revoked an average of only sixty-six doctors' licenses annually in the United States, even though incidents of careless and incompetent medical treatment are known to almost every physician and many patients.

As with many professional and industrial groups, the various bodies that police medicine have been created by or dominated by the profession that is to be policed. Advocates of regulatory reform say medicine's disciplinary bodies have remained weak because of the professional veil of silence that commonly shields serious incidents from outside attention, and because of the difficulty of getting patients to complain and testify against their doctors.

Lately more attention has been focused on the deficiencies of medical practice as the result of two forces. One is the growing involvement of the federal government in paying for health services. The other is the rise of the consumer movement which has stimulated activists, including conscientious doctors, to seek and disclose hitherto obscure information.

YOUR DOCTOR IS CRAMMING [3]

It wasn't all rest and relaxation for Dr. Bernard B. Zamostien as he recovered from a recent gall-bladder operation. In fact, he spent more time than usual studying the most recent advances in such things as thyroid and gynecologic problems, heart disease, immunology, and childhood ailments.

And for good reason. . . . Zamostien faces a challenge to his pride and ego, and a test of his competence as a doctor. He is a board-certified family physician, and along with more than 1,400 others he will take the first mandatory recertification exam ever required by a medical specialty in the United States.

"I don't relish taking the darn thing," Zamostien concedes. "If I flunk my recertification, I'm not going to lose my practice. But it will hurt my ego. I wouldn't want to explain to a patient in 1978 why my diploma only says [it is good] up to 1977."

Chart Reviews

Zamostien doesn't expect to flunk; he has kept up on the ever-changing ways of medicine. But all doctors certified as family-medicine specialists—there are now more than 8,700—must take a recertification test every six years. This exam —depending on your view—encourages or forces these doctors to keep current. And, says Zamostien, "the ultimate advantage is to the patient."

The family-physician recertification is designed to see how well physicians have kept up. All recertifications will

[3] Article by Patrick Young, staff correspondent. *National Observer.* p 6. O. 30, '76. Reprinted with permission of The National Observer. © Dow Jones & Company, Inc. 1976. All Rights Reserved.

be listed in the *Directory of Medical Specialties*. To take the test, eligible physicians must show three hundred hours of continuing medical education over the past six years. The test itself consists of a review of the doctor's patient charts and a written four-and-one-half-hour exam.

The doctors taking the exam . . . [in October 1976] completed their chart reviews. Each selected twenty of his patients' records, four each from five disease categories. Then he described the records and answered a series of questions designed to determine how well he treated these patients. Five percent of the doctors then were selected at random and asked to send copies of the records they had described in writing with all identification of the patients removed, so the accuracy of their answers could be checked by the recertification board. As for the written exam, says Zamostien, "There's not much you can do from a point of cramming. It's what you've been doing over the last six years."

New Material

The recertification of specialists and the relicensing of all physicians is a very controversial topic in the great debate over the quality of the nation's health care. Medical advances come in quantum leaps, piling one on another at a mind-boggling pace. Half the questions on Zamostien's exam will cover material so new they couldn't have been asked six years ago.

Until recently, a license to practice and a certificate as a specialist—surgeon, pediatrician, internist, etc.—were good essentially for life. But the consumer movement and an upsurge of malpractice suits have struck medicine, raising questions as to whether physicians are keeping properly informed and if greater efforts are needed to weed out incompetents.

Kennedy Bill

"Recertification and relicensing are the wave of the future," says Herbert Denenberg, former Pennsylvania insur-

ance commissioner and now a syndicated consumer col-
umnist. "It never made any sense to give a license for a
lifetime."

The government's medical-malpractice commission recommended in 1973 that all physicians and dentists be
relicensed periodically. Twelve states now require osteopathic physicians to show a certain number of hours of continuing medical education to be relicensed; eighteen states
have passed, but not all have implemented, such laws for
medical doctors. And Senator Edward Kennedy [Democrat,
Massachusetts] has twice introduced a bill requiring the
relicensing of physicians at least every six years by all states.

"If the federal government is going to buy services
through Medicare and Medicaid, we ought to be certain
we're buying good services," says a Kennedy aide. "We
shouldn't buy shoddy airplanes and we shouldn't buy
shoddy health care."

Although only the American Board of Family Practice
requires recertification for all its specialists, the other
twenty-one medical specialties have endorsed the retesting
principle. Three surgical specialties—general, thoracic, and
colon and rectal—require doctors certified after September
1, 1975, to be recertified every ten years. The rest plan
voluntary-recertification programs.

"Subtle Pressure"

Critics contend voluntary recertification is meaningless,
since only competent physicians will take the tests. But Dr.
Robert C. Derbyshire of Santa Fe, who led the successful
fight in New Mexico for relicensing requirements, disagrees.
He notes that all recertifications will be listed in the *Directory of Medical Specialties.*

"If I want to refer a patient to an internist in Los Angeles and I see one is recertified and one is not, I'll lean to
the one who is," Derbyshire says. "It's a subtle form of pressure."

But mandatory recertification and relicensing draw angry criticisms from many physicians who see themselves be-

ing singled out unjustly. "They are based on the premise that the exceptional doctor will keep abreast and all the rest have to have a degree of arm twisting to keep up," says Dr. Sanford Marcus of San Francisco, president of the American Union of Physicians. "There is a connotation there I don't like. If the assumption is that a doctor is going to let down all his excellence, I think the burden of proof is on the other side."

How He Keeps Up

Keeping abreast of medical developments, by one estimate, requires the equivalent of three months of forty-hour weeks each year. And a look at Zamostien's schedule provides a look at how one physician keeps current while serving the medical needs of some four thousand families.

Each week he scans about fifteen medical journals. In addition he takes short courses given at local, state, and national medical meetings, and at local hospitals and medical schools. In November he'll attend a day of lectures on recent advances in pediatrics, hemotology, immunology, rheumatology, obstetrics, and gynecology. Last year he attended a two-and-a-half-day refresher course in family medicine at Jefferson Medical College here [in Philadelphia].

Educational Questions

As an attending physician at Albert Einstein Medical Center [Temple University], Zamostien is required to attend 50 percent of the weekly "grand rounds" held ten months a year. At each a specific case or medical problem is presented and discussed. In the past six years, he has gained nearly one thousand hours in continuing-medical-education credits.

He also teaches occasional courses at Jefferson Medical College and works with third-year medical students from Temple University Medical School at Albert Einstein. The students' questions can be an education in themselves. "You know what you have to go home and look up," Zamostien says.

Buttressed by all this, Zamostien confronts his recertification with confidence and the feeling that it is good for both physicians and patients. "I don't think that test is the answer to being a great doctor, but it is definitely a step forward," he says. "And it does get rid of this idea that doctors just sit around on their butts and go to the bank."

HOW NURSES RATE HOSPITAL CARE [4]

It may seem a strange principle to enunciate as the very first requirement in a hospital that it should do the sick no harm. —Florence Nightingale.

That basic requirement is as valid today as it was in the nineteenth century, and few are in a better position to judge how well it is being met than Florence Nightingale's successors. Caring for patients long after staff doctors have made their daily rounds, nurses see hospitals at their very best moments—and their worst. For this reason the professional journal *Nursing77* (circulation: 400,000) asked its readers just what they think of the quality of care in the hospitals, nursing homes and other institutions employing them. The results add up to a disturbing diagnosis: in the opinion of the majority of the nurses who replied, health care in general deserves a grade no better than a low B.

More than ten thousand readers answered the seventy-eight multiple-choice questions, and *Nursing* says that well over two hundred were so "wound up" by the issues raised that they sent along letters detailing their complaints. Jean MacVicar, director of hospital nursing services of the National League for Nursing, notes that the strong reaction is "a sad commentary, but maybe we had to hit bottom before we decided to do something." Anne Zimmerman, president of the American Nurses' Association, concedes that people may find the report "unsettling," but is pleased nurses are finally speaking out. Says she: "The nurse is, after all, the patient's advocate."

    [4] Article from *Time.* 109:73. Ja. 17, '77. Reprinted by permission from *Time*, The Weekly Newsmagazine; copyright Time Inc. 1977.

Highlights of the survey:

☐ Fully 38 percent of the nurses said they would not, if they had a choice, be treated at their own hospitals. Wrote one: "All I have to say is, 'Dear God, may I never have to be a patient.'" As expected, many of the nays came from those employed by nursing homes, already the subject of widespread criticism. But there was also a surprising number of negative responses from small (under-200-bed) hospitals, traditionally thought to be the models of tender, loving care. Reported a nurse from one of these vest-pocket institutions: "Our emergency room has been known to call in a certain dentist for some cases when they can't reach an M.D."

☐ The nurses generally had high regard for the medical skills of their doctor colleagues; 28 percent considered the doctors excellent and 53 percent good, about the same rating they had for their fellow nurses' performance. But they were far less enthusiastic about the level of psychological support that the doctors give the sick; as many as 77 percent of the nurses assessed the doctors' performance in that area as either fair or poor. The most startling figure involved fatal accidents: 42 percent of the nurses said they knew of deaths that could be attributed to doctors' mistakes; 15 percent noted that they had witnessed such tragedies more than once. In her hospital, one nurse reported, a general surgeon lost eight patients over eight years through sheer ineptness. She added, "A psychiatrist on staff said that he was out to destroy himself."

☐ The nurses were considerably less harsh on themselves: 18 percent knew of deaths that had been caused by nursing errors and 4 percent admitted they had themselves made mistakes that might have led to patients' deaths. One nurse who let a critically ill man accidentally—and fatally—disconnect himself from a respirator wrote, "That was three years ago and I still can't get it out of my mind."

☐ Many nurses griped about their increasing load of paper work. Snapped one: "If I'd wanted to get secretary's bottom I could have stayed at my old job." Others said that personnel shortages were forcing them to neglect patients' needs. But what especially irked them was the indifference of doctors to nurses' opinions about patients. As one nurse put it, "Sometimes you wonder why you have to make the rounds with an M.D. when he totally ignores your questions and/or your suggestions."

As might be expected, the survey is running into some flak. Since it expresses only the views of nurses who took the trouble to fill out and mail the questionnaire, it may well be biased in favor of those eager to air complaints. Commenting on the nurses' reluctance to seek care in their own institutions, American Hospital Association President J. Alexander McMahon cracked: "It reminds me of the joke, 'Any country club that would admit me, I wouldn't want to join.'" As for himself, he insisted, "I would have no hesitation in being admitted to any hospital in the United States." That may well be. Yet so critical a report from within the medical profession will surely have repercussions, possibly for the good. Coming at a time of rising public concern over the quality and cost (a record $140 billion in fiscal 1976) of medical care, it will give reformers new arguments in their demands for major improvements in the US health system.

II. THE QUESTION OF COSTS

EDITOR'S INTRODUCTION

Medical care in America today is big business. It employs 4.8 million people and is therefore one of the largest industries in the nation. Only manufacturing and the wholesale and retail trade employ more people.

Yet the medical-care industry is not a very competitive one. Doctors and hospitals, for example, don't compete for business by giving more for less (or less for less). But then, the average consumer of medical services probably does not want them to. For one thing, sick patients want help—at any cost; for another, most patients do not pay that cost directly. Third parties—private insurance companies, Medicare, and Medicaid—pay about 90 percent of all hospital bills. Thus, to consumers, the idea of pressing hospitals to cut costs does not seem terribly urgent—especially when the first priority is getting well.

This section opens with an article from *Newsweek*, "Health-Cost Crisis," that provides an overview of the problem of medical care costs. The second article, "Paying the Doctor," by Christine E. Bishop, assistant professor of economics at Boston University, points out some of the reasons for the sharp rise in physicians' fees over the past decade. Another selection from *Newsweek* follows. Written by Dr. Maurice Fox, a practitioner of internal medicine, it rebuts the charges that doctors make too much money and fail to listen to their patients' complaints.

Does the profit motive impede the delivery of low-cost medical care? The next article, written by James L. Goddard, former commissioner of the United States Food and Drug Administration, now chairman of the board of a drug and chemical firm, and taken from *Scientific American*, asserts that the costs of drugs, medical supplies, and equipment add enormously to the expense of medical care. The section concludes with a *U.S. News & World Report* article on the cost of technology by associate editor Abigail Trafford Brett, who questions whether the increased costs resulting from the increased use of expensive techniques are justified in terms of meaningful gains for the patients concerned. She also points up the growing problem of the misuse of technology.

HEALTH-COST CRISIS [1]

☐ Juanita and Roy Tomblinson of Denver took their disabled son from doctor to doctor and clinic to clinic for treatment of cerebral palsy. Batteries of tests, a series of corrective operations and years of physical therapy exhausted their medical insurance and left the couple with $10,000 worth of bills to pay.

☐ Lucy and Kenneth Knight of Santa Monica, California, lived a comfortable life until sickness struck. Knight suffered a devastating heart attack and underwent cardiac surgery. Then his wife developed breast cancer and had two operations. The Knights were forced to take out loans to help pay nearly $9,000 of costs not covered by their health insurance.

☐ Dr. Lowell Baker, a Houston Health Department physician, had not been on the city payroll long enough for full insurance-coverage when he suffered a coronary. He wiped out his savings and went into debt to pay nearly $15,000 in hospital and doctor bills.

These cases make dramatically plain just how expensive medical care in the United States can be. . . . Expenditures have been rising like the line on a pneumonia patient's fever chart. Major health-care costs jumped to $93 billion during the course of the last fiscal year [1976] and this figure did not include the cost of dentistry and such other expenses as nursing and home care. Health-care costs have risen about 50 percent faster than have other items on the

[1] From article by Matt Clark and others, staff writers. *Newsweek*. 89:84+. My. 9, '77. Copyright 1977 by Newsweek, Inc. Reprinted by permission.

consumer price index. The nation's total health bill is increasing by a staggering $1 billion a month over the corresponding month last year and the end of the rise is not yet in sight: it is anticipated that the cost will double in the next five years—to an estimated $280 billion.

Concern about the surge in costs has taken on a new urgency in recent years because of the federal government's growing part in providing health care. The Medicare program for the elderly will cost the United States $22 billion this fiscal year and the federal share of the Medicaid program for the poor will be $10 billion.

At the same time, evidence of waste, mismanagement and outright fraud in Medicare and Medicaid has led to serious doubts about the role the federal government should play in the nation's health care. "It is all too apparent," says a report of the Council on Wage and Price Stability, "that the federal government, instead of being part of the solution, is part of the problem of rising health-care costs."

Fraud and abuse are only a small part of the total picture. Health-care costs have gotten out of hand for a score of complex reasons, and the prognosis for getting them in check is, as the doctors say, guarded at best. Some of the increase is part of the current inflation rampant throughout the nation's economy. Additional impetus for rising costs has come from the vastly expanding—and expensive—technology that has made medicine more of a science and less of an art in recent years and produced dramatic advances in diagnosis and treatment.

Health insurance has made medical care more available —and stimulated greater demand for health service. In New York City alone, there were 50 million Medicaid claims paid in 1976. Blue Cross, Blue Shield and a multiplicity of private health insurance programs now cover nearly 80 percent of the nation's medical bill, compared with only 37 percent in 1950. A General Motors executive says that his firm's outlay for health insurance contributes more to the cost of a car than does the price of the steel.

Ordinarily, prices would be expected to rise when the

demand for services exceeds the supply. But one peculiarity of US medical care is that the law of supply and demand doesn't apply. Health-care facilities, including hospitals and the doctors who work in them, have expanded in size and number apace with demand. Yet, there are still further increases in cost. "I find it absolutely mind-boggling," said John J. O'Connell, a vice president of Bethlehem Steel, "that an industry this size operates in our economy almost completely immune to the forces most basic to the economy."

The average patient stands in awe of the medical profession and willingly acquiesces to the role of passive participant in the health-care process. "Americans canonize doctors," says one Blue Cross official. "They put more emphasis on health care, and they like their doctors in Cadillacs instead of Volkswagens." And since insurance is apt to pay for much of the patient's care, neither he nor the doctor is likely to be very concerned about the costs.

Three or Four Tests

The current crisis in malpractice suits also has prompted doctors to practice "defensive medicine," ordering up three or four tests or X-rays in order to cover themselves, when only one would do. A survey reported by the Journal of the American Medical Association disclosed that three out of four physicians call for extra tests.

Physicians' fees account for almost 20 percent of health-care costs and they have risen at the rate of more than 11 percent. However, there are wide variations in physicians' costs because doctors traditionally have based their charges on what the traffic will bear. In New York, a gall-bladder removal is $1,000; in Findley, Ohio, the same operation costs $200.

Doctors argue that inflation has victimized them along with their patients. "Everything I buy costs more," says Dr. Julius H. Jacobson II, a vascular surgeon at New York's Mount Sinai Hospital. "I just bought a pair of bandage scissors for $42 that used to cost $7."

Hospitals account for 40 percent of the nation's health-care expenditure. And because the hospital is the doctor's workshop, many experts believe physicians must share much of the responsibility for rising hospital costs. "The world's greatest hospital manager could lower costs by maybe 10 percent," says Dr. Samuel P. Martin III of the University of Pennsylvania's National Health Care Management Center, "but 85 percent of utilization [of hospitals] is in the hands of the doctors."

A Waving of Wands

Hospitals purchase much of their equipment to cater to the doctor's needs, or what the doctor perceives as his patient's needs. Coronary intensive-care units, heart-lung machines, automated blood analyzers and CAT [computerized axial tomography] scanners, X-ray devices that provide a cross-sectional picture of the body, have added enormously to improved medical care. But they have also increased costs. A CAT scanner may sell for $600,000 or more and it costs $180,000 a year to maintain and equip an open-heart surgery team.

There is also evidence that the proliferation of expensive technology has led to vast waste and duplication of facilities. In many communities, for example, cardiac-surgery teams are not kept busy enough to maintain their skills because there are simply too many of them for the number of patients requiring such surgery. "I think that doctors have to realize that they cannot continue to wave wands," HEW Secretary Califano told Newsweek, "and order up sophisticated equipment and expensive capital additions to hospitals simply because it makes life a little easier for them."

The willy-nilly expansion of hospital facilities has led to "overbedding" and a substantial addition to the problem of health costs. Any empty bed costs money because a hospital must still maintain the same facilities and staff that would be required if it were to be filled. On any given day, according to one estimate, there are 100,000 empty hospital

beds in the United States, representing an annual loss to
the health industry of $2 billion.

Overbedding means wasteful duplication of facilities.
Owing to the drop in the nation's birth rate, many hospitals
have nearly empty obstetrical units. In the Delaware Valley, which encompasses eight counties around Philadelphia,
there are sixty-two hospitals that offer pediatric services and
the average occupancy for each is only 50 percent.

In addition, hospital accounting procedures often seem
unrelated to conventional business practice. The charge for
a room covers expenses such as housekeeping, food, nursing, heat and power that are not itemized on a patient's bill.
Charges for drugs and other items also are inflated to cover
such overhead expenses as operating a social service department. An audit in Georgia, for instance, found some hospitals that were charging $40 to $50 for a bottle of aspirin
and $35 for a bottle of Listerine.

A Day or Two Longer

Insurance companies such as Blue Cross compound the
problem because they reimburse hospitals for a patient's
care on a flat daily rate, based on the average charges for all
patients treated. The first few days in a hospital are the
most expensive because that's when the lab tests and surgical procedures are done, and the last days the cheapest as
the patient recovers. Since the reimbursement rate is the
same each day, the incentive is to keep patients a day or
two longer than necessary to avoid losing money in difficult
cases.

According to experts, a reduction of one day in the current average stay of seven days in the hospital would save
$2 billion a year. One way to get around the flat per diem
problem, which will be tested in New Jersey, would be to
reimburse hospitals a set amount depending on the particular diagnosis, regardless of how long the patient stays. For
a tonsillectomy a hospital might get $400 while it might re-
ceive $10,000 more for complicated open-heart surgery.

Gradually, other solutions are being tried to curb rising

health-care costs. One method advocated by many health planners is the health maintenance organization, a group of doctors working on a salaried, rather than fee-for-service basis. For a monthly premium, all of a patient's medical needs are supplied. Because the doctors work on a salary, they have no incentive to provide unnecessary services. Numerous studies have shown that patients under successful prepaid groups spend fewer days in the hospital than those belonging to indemnity programs like Blue Cross.

Getting a Second Opinion

Health insurance plans have begun to move against unnecessary surgery and hospitalization by encouraging—and paying for—consultation for second opinions when operations are recommended. One recent study in New York City showed that consultants disagreed with the need for surgery in 17 percent of cases. Consequently, Blue Shield of New York, and insurers in several other states, now pay for second opinions.

Industry, which underwrites an increasing share of the health bill, is also beginning to take initiatives to hold down costs. Motorola, Inc., in Phoenix, Arizona, which pays directly for the care received by 43,000 employees, demanded that three of the city's hospitals divulge financial records when the company noted a 56 percent rise in hospital costs in a single year. Eventually, the company forced the hospitals into negotiations leading to cost-cutting reforms.

Perhaps the greatest impact on rising health-care costs will be made by enforcement of the 1974 National Health Planning and Resources Development Act. A top priority item in the Administration's plans to curtail health costs, the law is only now beginning to be implemented. It requires that hospitals and nursing homes prove that they have a definite need for building additional facilities or buying new equipment—and thus avoid wasteful duplication. Any institutions that go ahead without approval for new construction or purchasing will not be reimbursed by the federal Medicare and Medicaid programs. Such measures, say health experts, will not by themselves halt the skyrocketing cost of medical care in the United States. But they are a vitally needed first step—taken none too soon.

PAYING THE DOCTOR [2]

The availability and quality of medical care are . . . affected by the way physicians are paid in our health-care system. While a significant proportion of their work is performed in hospitals, most physicians are not paid by these health institutions, but by their patients, on a fee-for-service basis. Physicians earn more if they perform more fee-generating services, and they typically work long hours: nonfederal physicians in office practice worked an average of 49.9 hours per week in 1974.

They also earn more if fees rise. For most goods and services, price directly influences the consumer's decision; he or she evaluates carefully whether the item is worth its price, and high prices are likely to discourage purchases. The prices of physician services do not play this role for many consumers, who are covered by private health insurance or by government health programs (Medicare and Medicaid) for in-hospital physician care and, increasingly, for some outpatient care as well. Physicians have apparently been able to raise fees without reducing the demand for their services or affecting the financial situation of individual patients, since third parties (insurance companies and government agencies) pay the bills.

Physician fees have been one of the most rapidly rising components of the consumer price index (CPI), increasing 70.8 percent between 1965 and 1974, while the consumer price index as a whole rose 56.3 percent. (The recent rate of change in fees has been somewhat less than the rate of change of the CPI). Of course, physicians expect to recover

[2] From "Health Employment and the Nation's Health," by Christine E. Bishop, assistant professor of economics, Boston University. *Current History.* 72:208–9. My./Je. '77. Copyright © 1977 by Current History, Inc. Reprinted by permission.

their expenses for office equipment, personnel, and supplies, and to make a net income for themselves. That physician incomes are high is to be expected for workers who make such a large time and money investment in their training; the average net income for nonfederal physicians in office-based practice was $51,224 in 1974. However, studies have found that the investment in medical education produces a rate of return significantly higher than other training and financial investments an individual might make; estimates for the rate of return to medical education range from 15 percent to 18 percent. High incomes mean that subsidies to induce physicians to practice in areas or specialties where they are most needed are unlikely to be effective, since physicians can apparently do well in most of the locations or specialties they might choose. Rapidly rising fees feed health-cost inflation, and physician fees are clearly a significant component of rising national health expenditures.

Plans and programs to improve the availability and quality of health care in this country and to control its total cost may involve changes in the way physicians are paid. Under a prepaid group practice arrangement, for example, individuals pay the group practice organization a premium or capitation which covers all health care for a year. If physicians, who make most decisions about patient care, choose less costly modes of care when appropriate (for example outpatient care instead of in-hospital treatment for certain conditions) and avoid tests and procedures that have only marginal value for patient health, savings can be returned to the organization for distribution to physicians and/or the membership. Physicians are thus not paid for doing more to patients, but are rewarded for saving costs and maintaining member health (hence the term "health maintenance organization," or "HMOs," which applies to both prepaid group practice and fee-for-service foundations for medical care). [For additional information, see Section VI, below.] Public policy has encouraged the growth of prepaid group practice, and any comprehensive national health insurance program may be expected to further reinforce any cost-saving aspects of this practice. It has been argued that physicians will not work as long hours for salaries or group rewards as they work for individual fees; this may prove true, but is less of a cause for concern in light of our expanding physician supply.

WHY PEOPLE ARE MAD AT DOCTORS [3]

These days, a physician can't go to any sort of social gathering without being surrounded by people who want desperately to talk about doctors and money. First, they describe with pride the achievements of a son or nephew whose brilliance enabled him to get into medical school. Next, just a word or two about their own symptoms—not enough to be overbearing. Then, having demonstrated a fundamental sympathy with your life's work, the mood changes and they begin to purge themselves of deeply felt grievances. They express disappointment, hurt, resentment and self-righteous anger. They are mad as hell at doctors.

The major criticisms I hear are that doctors don't listen sufficiently to patients' complaints, and that doctors make too much money.

The first is a profoundly serious criticism, and one hears it so often that there must be some substance to it. But what does the patient mean when he says "the doctor doesn't listen"? Most of the time, the patient means that the doctor does not spend enough time with him and does not provide enough of the "caring" functions of doctoring.

I submit it is true that some physicians see too many patients. I don't think anyone can provide quality care when only five minutes or so are spent with a patient, unless all the complaints are trivial (known in the trade as "colds and clap"). Most high-quality internists I know, with large practices of significantly ill patients, are stretched near the breaking point with thirty patients per ten- to

[3] Article by Dr. Maurice Fox, who practices internal medicine in Palo Alto, California. *Newsweek*. 89:4. Ja. 10, '77. Copyright 1977 by Newsweek, Inc. Reprinted by permission.

twelve-hour day. Working at this pace, the physician is hard-pressed to deal with his patients' emotional needs as well as their medical requirements.

Talking to Patients

Many patients go to doctors with no real bodily ills, but are depressed and fearful. Their lives may be painful, empty and disappointing. Often the physician can do little to make these patients feel better. When all the examinations fail to turn up an organic abnormality, the patient is often frustrated and angry. The sensitive physician can relieve anxiety and guilt by reassuring the patient that he knows that he, the patient, feels terrible, but that medicine has no means at present to cure this kind of suffering. Sick patients also are always afraid and uncomfortable and want to feel their physician is concerned with their personal welfare as well as with the diagnosis. Most physicians know this need has to be met if the patient is to be satisfied. All this takes time. So why doesn't the physician have enough time to provide these comforts and "talk to patients"?

Most of the time, he does. Sometimes no amount of talking or caring can improve a particularly desperate situation. Sometimes the patients' demands are excessive. There are a number of patients who, given unlimited access, would use up all the working hours of this country's physicians and leave most of the population in the waiting room. With the isolation of urban American society and the fragmentation of multigeneration families, there may be no one to whom one can carry one's troubles. So people go to doctors to buy a little love and attention. This is a misuse of physicians' time.

Money and Medicine

The other complaint—that doctors make too much money—also bears scrutiny. Doctors are fairly well paid in this country, but when one considers the hours and the burdens, they earn their income. Many in business and other professions are paid more for less work. Some doctors make an awful lot of money, but they don't make it by talking to patients. And that's where the issues of doctors, money and talk come together.

The fact is that the primary physician, the talking and caring doctor, is not paid much for talking and caring. Somehow or other, a system of physician compensation has developed in this country so that the less a doctor talks to you and the more he does to you the more he is paid. The radiologist who looks at your X-rays, and may never even see you, the pathologist who looks at pieces cut out of you (biopsies), the surgeon and anesthesiologist who work on you while you are asleep—all these physicians earn more than those who deal with you awake and have to "talk to you." This is because physicians are much more highly paid for "procedures" than for such services as treating diabetes and heart disease.

Society's willingness to place much more value on the time of a physician (or dentist or podiatrist) who does a procedure than on the time of the physician who provides a medical service is responsible for many of the problems of our health-care system. Is it really in society's best interest that surgeons earn so much more money than pediatricians? A pediatrician, who cares for the health of the coming generation, and, by advising parents, plays a major role in the emotional health of the young, earns on the average less than half as much as a surgeon.

Is that what this service is truly worth to society? It is not unusual to find that a woman who prepaid $1,200 to have her face lifted is outraged when her internist submits a bill for $200 for spending from 1 to 3 A.M. with her in the coronary-care unit to pull her through her heart attack. Does she really value her appearance that much more than her life? The cost of several new procedures, such as total hip replacement and coronary bypass, is so high that with wide application the whole health insurance structure could be threatened. Shouldn't we start paying attention to these problems now, before they reach crisis proportions?

Toward Better Care

It is probably true that since compensation is so much higher for procedures than for medical services, more procedures tend to get done. This is not because the physician is dishonest, but because the "style" of practice tends to lean toward more doing and less talking. Many patients demand more tests and procedures, thinking this gets them better medical care. Often, the best service the well-trained physician can offer a patient is to advise that nothing can be done. This is frequently not understood and not appreciated by the patient.

If some doctors make too much money, they are very rarely the primary physicians, unless they are seeing too many patients. I tell my cocktail-party friends that if they want their physician to spend more time listening and talking to them, then they should respect the value of the service he renders by talking to them and thinking about them, just as much as they respect the time he spends doing something to them.

COSTLY DRUGS AND SUPPLIES [4]

In this article I shall be concerned with the substantial fraction of the total medical care bill that supports the "medical business": the $11 billion expended for drugs, medical supplies and equipment. To put the $11 billion in perspective, it is roughly a third of what Americans spent in 1972 on new automobiles.

In the field of ethical pharmaceuticals—drugs sold only on prescription—there are some 22,000 trade-name products in the marketplace. In the field of devices, medical equipment and supplies, there is no reliable estimate of the num-

[4] Article entitled "The Medical Business," by Dr. James L. Goddard, former commissioner of the U.S. Food and Drug Administration, currently chairman of board of Ormont Drug and Chemical Company. *Scientific American.* 229:161–6. S. '73. Copyright © 1973 by Scientific American, Inc. Reprinted by permission. All rights reserved.

ber of products manufactured but it almost certainly exceeds 20,000. They range from cotton balls, sutures and tongue depressors to $100,000 blood-analysis machines that can measure twelve components in a blood sample at the rate of sixty samples per hour. There are more differences than similarities between the pharmaceutical industry and the industries involved in the production of devices, medical supplies and equipment. Here are some of the major differences.

Perhaps the most significant difference is the way in which the consumer pays for the products involved. Consumers paid directly 85 percent of the more than $6 billion spent at retail for 1.5 billion drug prescriptions filled in 1971. In contrast some mode of indirect payment was involved for 84 percent of the consumable supplies and equipment used during illnesses in the same year. Prosthetic devices, including eyeglasses, which are paid for directly, accounted for the remaining 16 percent. Supplies are said to be paid for indirectly when they are part of a consolidated bill presented by a hospital or clinic or when they are part of a bill paid by an insurance carrier or other third party. In either case the patient is usually unaware of the details.

A corollary of the mode of payment leads to the second major difference between the drug houses and the makers of medical supplies: the degree of product visibility. The general public is aware of and concerned about such issues as the safety of oral contraceptives, price-fixing in antibiotics and the debate over brand-name versus generic-name prescription writing. The public has little or no interest, however, in such matters as proof of safety and effectiveness of equipment used for patient care or the unnecessary duplication of costly equipment by hospitals located in the same area. One thinks, for example, of the fad for installing hyperbaric chambers in hospital operating rooms in the mid-1960s. Costing upward of $100,000 per installation, their value to the patient undergoing surgery now appears marginal.

Product visibility, or lack of it, helps to explain the third major difference between the part of the industry that produces drugs and the part that produces supplies and equipment. Whereas the government subjects drug makers to heavy regulation, it has only recently begun to regulate the makers of medical supplies and equipment.

The fourth major difference between the two parts of the industry is in profitability. The pharmaceutical houses outperform all other major American industries in net profit after taxes as a percent of stockholders' equity. The drug companies regularly show a return of about 18 percent, a figure two thirds higher than the average rate of return for all manufacturing concerns in the decade 1960–1970. Although the consolidated data are not available for direct comparison, it is evident from the annual reports of the major companies in the medical supplies and equipment business that their rates of return are closer to the industrial average of 11 percent than to the drug companies' 18 percent. These, then, are the two major segments of the medical business: one highly visible, highly profitable and highly controversial, the other almost hidden from view, returning only average profits and making few "waves." Let us now take a closer look at the two segments.

The Pharmaceutical Industry

The pharmaceutical industry manufactures two major classes of products: proprietary drugs sold freely over the counter and ethical drugs, which require a prescription. Ethical pharmaceuticals are further subdivided into brand-name and generic products. The former are patented products manufactured by the larger companies; the latter are substances on which the patent has usually expired and that bear a uniform chemical name regardless of the source.

In 1971, according to surveys conducted by the magazine *Drug Topics*, the dollar volume of all packaged medicines sold at retail without a prescription was $2.9 billion. Of this total, cough and cold "remedies" accounted for $619 million, headache nostrums for $600 million and mouthwashes and gargles for $240 million. Many observers question the desirability of this traffic in drugs that are mostly marginal in their effectiveness. Although they are heavily advertised as being capable of relieving and even curing various target ailments, the claims are rarely supported by objective studies. The Federal Trade Commission has begun to look closely at the curative claims made for these over-the-counter drugs in television and newspaper advertisements.

Meanwhile the prescription drug industry is enjoying an unbroken rise in sales. The value of ethical-drug shipments in 1971 was $4.11 billion, an increase of more than 100 percent in ten years, with no leveling off in sight. If Congress were to enact some kind of comprehensive national health insurance plan that would include payment for prescription drugs, total sales could jump from 20 to 25 percent almost overnight. . . .

It is estimated that the ethical-drug houses currently spend $1.2 billion per year on advertising and promotion. This represents about $1 in every $4 they receive for their products at wholesale and is nearly four times what they spend annually on research and development. Virtually none of the marketing expenditures are directed at the consumer who buys the product. They are directed at the physician who writes the prescription and at the pharmacist who, with increasing frequency, is in a position to select the brand when the prescription is written generically or when it allows him to substitute one brand for another.

Since the marketing costs come to about $4,000 per physician per year they are deemed excessive by many critics of the industry. The $1.2-billion figure includes the salaries of more than 21,000 "detail men," each of whom costs the industry an estimated $35,000 per year; their sole job is to make periodic calls on physicians, pharmacists and hospital purchasing agents to push their firm's products. Also included in the $1.2 billion are such costs as advertising in medical journals, exhibits at medical conventions, direct-mail pieces (including physicians' samples), seminars, educational films, brochures and the practice of allowing wholesalers, retailers and hospitals to return unsold merchandise for credit. How essential these expenditures are is a matter of judgment. That they add significantly to the nation's drug bill is undisputable.

During the past five years research costs in the pharmaceutical industry have averaged close to 6 percent of net sales, a figure comparable to that in other high-technology industries. In the same period the return on research investments, as measured by new products, has shown a steady decline. The decline followed the passage of the Kefauver-Harris amendments to the federal Food, Drug, and Cosmetic Act of 1962, which substantially increased the Food and Drug Administration's regulating authority with respect to the testing and marketing of new drugs. The peak for new chemical entities (63) was reached in 1959; the peaks for new combinations (253) and new dosage forms (109) had been reached a year earlier. By requiring that new drugs be efficacious as well as safe, the Kefauver-Harris amendments accelerated the decline in all three categories of new products. With 5,558 new products entering the marketplace between 1950 and 1962 the country needed not more combinations, new dosage forms and duplicate products but more effective drugs.

In spite of some predictions the amendments have not stifled drug research. The quest for new drugs continues apace. The total industry outlay for research and development exceeds $500 million per year, and the federal government spends $1.75 billion on drug testing alone.

Production costs in the pharmaceutical industry average a third of the manufacturer's sales dollar. The most significant portion of this expenditure, however, is related not to the cost of raw materials or to the manufacturing process itself but rather to the highly complex quality-control procedures required by federal law. More than eight thousand workers, 16 percent of the industry's work force, are engaged in quality control.

Profitability

Profitability has long been the hallmark of the pharmaceutical industry. Year after year the industry ranks first or second in after-tax income as a percentage of net worth. This profitability has been maintained by the drug industry even though drug prices have not climbed as rapidly as consumer prices in general. The drug industry has been able to limit price increases thanks in large part to the high degree of automatic control achieved in its manufacturing processes. At the same time the absence of price competition for most products has ensured continued high profits.

When the pharmaceutical industry is called on to defend its large profit margins, it responds that it is in a high-risk business in which vast sums are spent on research with little or no guarantee of return. Spokesmen for the drug industry often compare the search for new drugs with the drilling of wildcat wells in the oil industry. The fact is that during the past twenty-five years no major pharmaceutical house has been forced out of business. As one economist said in testimony before the Senate Select Committee on Small Business: "The high profitability reflects the absence of competition; the stability of profits demonstrates the absence of risk to investors. If risks were to exist, one would expect to see the high gains of some firms accompanied by occasional losses—to themselves or to others—but such evidence of risk is virtually nonexistent."

The industry's profitability has been maintained also in the face of rising government interest in and control of its activities. Federal interest was aroused in the era of Theodore Roosevelt, when the blatant claims of many makers of patent medicines led to calls for government regulation. Apart from the fact that the claims were often misleading and even dangerous, many of the nostrums contained opium derivatives, with the result that many people unwittingly became addicted to the drug. Harvey W. Wiley, a chemist in the Department of Agriculture, was one of the leaders in the effort to bring patent medicines under control. It was not until the publication of Upton Sinclair's novel *The Jungle*, however, that Congress responded by passing the Food and Drug Act of 1906. From this modest beginning the federal role in drug regulation has grown to its present level. In each instance drug legislation granting new authority was precipitated by some crisis affecting the consumer.

In 1938, for example, it was the elixir of sulfanilamide disaster, in which the use of ethylene glycol as a solvent by a chemist with the S. E. Massengill Company led to the death of more than one hundred persons, most of them small children. Congress swiftly enacted a law requiring that drugs be proved safe prior to marketing. Such legislation had been sought by the executive branch of the government each year since 1933, only to be beaten back each time in Congress through the efforts of the drug-industry lobby.

In 1961, when the thalidomide tragedy struck in Europe, Richardson-Merrell, Inc., a major US pharmaceutical manufacturer, had a new-drug application for thalidomide pending before the Food and Drug Administration. Thanks to the vigilance of Frances Oldham Kelsey, a physician and pharmacologist on the FDA staff, the application was held up and ultimately never issued. Congress again acted swiftly by passing the Kefauver-Harris amendments which provided the FDA with an entire range of new authorities, including the requirement that all new drugs must be proved not only safe but also effective before being allowed to enter the marketplace. The FDA was also empowered to require periodic reports from manufacturers; to require that ethical-drug advertising be honest, with sufficient balance to give the physician information about a drug's side effects and contraindications as well as its potential benefits; to require immediate reporting of any unusual side effects during development work, and to review all drugs marketed between 1938 and 1962 to determine their efficacy as well as their safety.

Some observers believe that the pharmaceutical industry is now overregulated and that bureaucratic interference with the industry has reached such a level that the American public is being denied certain drugs available overseas. The University of Chicago economist Milton Friedman has recently made this point forcefully, and with much publicity, by charging that FDA regulations are keeping important new drugs off the American market and that the United States is falling behind the rest of the world in the development of new drugs. Calling for repeal of the Kefauver-Harris amendments, Friedman pointed to the availability in Europe of two new drugs for heart patients, Practolol and Oxprenolol, as prime examples of why the present system should be changed.

Friedman's allegations were effectively refuted during recent Senate hearings by spokesmen from three organizations that rarely find themselves in total agreement about anything: the Food and Drug Administration, the American Medical Association and the Pharmaceutical Manufacturers Association. Spokesmen for these groups, along with a number of prominent heart and cancer specialists, made it quite clear that even though the United States has the most demanding requirements of any nation in the world, all safe and effective drugs, or their equivalents, are available here. (Practolol and Oxprenolol are not deemed safe.)

Manufacturers of Medical Supplies, Devices, and Equipment

The companies that manufacture medical supplies, devices and equipment might be termed the hidden, or at least the unknown, segment of the medical business. When the patient is billed for blood tests or X-rays, it probably does not occur to him that part of the fee is used to offset the purchase price of expensive analytical instruments or an X-ray camera. And who even cares that the doctor's bill must cover the cost of tongue depressors, Band-Aids, thermometers, disposable hypodermic syringes and the almost countless other impedimenta of medical practice?

In spite of their low profile, the companies that make these medical goods are enjoying the sharply rising expenditures on health care. For example, manufacturers of surgical dressings and instruments have annual sales of more than $500 million. This amount includes $163 million for adhesive tape, $127 million for compresses, gauze and other dressings, $88 million for elastic bandages and rolls containing plaster of Paris for making casts and $30 million for cotton balls. Sales of surgical instruments come to about $120 million per year.

Manufacturers of other kinds of medical supplies have annual sales of more than $2 billion. Sales are expected to reach $2.9 billion by 1975 and $4.2 billion by 1980. Products under this heading include anesthetics, parenteral solutions, syringes and needles, sutures, laboratory ware and reagents, thermometers, stethoscopes, sphygmomanometers, medical linen and X-ray supplies. (More square feet of photographic film are consumed in making X-rays than are used by the motion picture industry, which has recently led the Eastman Kodak Company to introduce a system for copying the standard 14-by-17-inch X-ray image on a "chip" about two inches square so that the silver in the original large negative can be recycled.)

The introduction of new technology, much of it made possible by solid-state electronics, has led to a sharp rise in the sales of medical and hospital equipment. The magazine *Electronics* predicts, for example, that sales will increase more than 50 percent between 1970 and 1975: from $530 million to $832 million. Sales of patient-monitoring systems will nearly triple in the same period: from $29 million to $80 million.

Sizable increases are also predicted for sales of such laboratory equipment as automatic clinical chemistry systems, blood-bank equipment, blood analyzers, chromatography systems, electrolyte-measuring instruments, automatic blood-cell counters, electron and light miscroscopes and spectrophotometers. Sales of these items, which were less than $200 million in 1968, may reach $380 million in 1975 and exceed $570 million in 1980, according to *Electronics*.

The use of new plastics and alloys has led to great advances in such surgical implants as artificial joints, bone plates, pins and arterial grafts. It is estimated that 100,000 arterial grafts will be inserted this year, along with 45,000 heart valves and 200,000 cerebrospinal-fluid shunts (mechanical devices for relieving excess aqueous pressure within the brain). It is estimated that 100,000 Americans are now equipped with electronic heart pacemakers and that 50,000 new installations will be made this year. More than three million women have now been fitted with intrauterine contraceptive devices (IUDs) in the form of rings, coils, loops, bows, springs and spirals.

During the remainder of the decade one can expect major progress in the development of assistive, prosthetic and corrective devices, such as "radar" aids for the blind and artificial larynxes. Sales of devices in this category are expected to reach $640 million by 1975 and $890 million by 1980.

Need for Adequate Controls

Many observers believe the medical-supply industry is in the same position as the drug industry was in before the enactment of the 1938 legislation. There has been an enormous proliferation of medical devices (a recent FDA [Food and Drug Administration] survey counted 12,000 devices made by 1,100 companies), but no federal agency has yet been given the responsibility for determining either their safety or their efficacy. The International Organization for Standardization has been pressing its member countries to exercise greater control over devices with the greatest potential for doing harm, particularly surgical implants. At the same time the FDA has been asking Congress to increase its control over the manufacture and sale of medical devices of all kinds.

In recent testimony before a congressional subcommittee the then Acting FDA Commissioner Sherwin Gardner noted that under the limited powers granted the agency in 1938 most of its effort, until recently at least, had been devoted to removing obviously dangerous products from the market and controlling the promotion of "quack type" de-

vices. "Because existing law imposes no statutory requirements for FDA to review the safety and effectiveness of medical devices prior to marketing," Gardner testified, "FDA
has the burden of proof and must accumulate evidence sufficient to assure that it can sustain a court action."

An indication of the seriousness of the problem is that,
even with such limited powers, the FDA in the first three
months of this year [1973] seized more than 300 devices,
ordered the recall of 35 different kinds of device (including
several hundred heart pacemakers) and issued more than
1,800 advisory opinions (letters of warning or caution to
manufacturers). A bill that is currently before Congress
would enable the agency to require all manufacturers of
medical devices to be registered with the FDA, to disclose
all complaints received, to maintain records and submit reports (including clinical studies of safety and efficacy)
and to recall, replace or repair defective devices. One would
hope that adequate control legislation will for once in this
country be enacted on its merits and not in response to a
tragedy.

THE COST OF TECHNOLOGY [5]

Reprinted from *U.S. News & World Report*.

The growing power and sophistication of technology is
rapidly overhauling the practice of medicine to an extent
realized by few Americans.

Never have doctors been able to do so much to thwart
the course of disease—and rarely have issues been so complex, or so disturbing. Gradually the magic of healing has
been replaced by the mystique of science.

Physicians and patients alike await test results with the
same anticipation as ancients consulting the oracles. Gone
are the black bag of pills and the house call. Now it is the
hospital—the medical repository of space-age technology—
that issues judgment on human life and death.

[5] From "New Medical Technology: Is It Worth the Price?" by A. T. Brett, associate editor. *U.S. News & World Report.* 82:43–5. My. 23, '77.

In the stainless-steel cocoon of the intensive-care unit, a variety of bewildering machines take over functions of the heart, lung, kidney, bowel. They breathe, pump blood, consume fluids, check pulse rates and brain waves. They literally live for the disabled patient. . . .

Longer Life Expectancy

Today more lives are being saved than ever before. More conditions can be treated successfully. Life expectancy is longer today than it was ten years ago, and infant mortality is down.

But there is a price. New techniques are so powerful that sometimes they can be worse than the disease, particularly for certain cancer and coronary patients.

Technology may prolong survival but not meaningful life. There is the specter of a Karen Quinlan, saved by technology, but doomed to live as a vegetable.

Misuse of technology by physicians is a growing problem. Charges are heard that unnecessary tests and surgery often are performed.

In addition, the tripling of health costs in the last decade is directly related to the increased use of expensive techniques.

No one doubts that medicine's technological revolution is here to stay. But the question is being asked: How much technology is enough? From Dr. Niall P. Macallister, director of the surgical intensive-care unit at Johns Hopkins Hospital in Baltimore, comes this warning: "Technology is an expensive dray horse dragging us along at one hundred miles an hour—but where are we going?"

Many physicians fear that the current reaction against technology will stall the progress of medical science just when it's beginning to get somewhere in treating many diseases. At the same time, they say, the mechanization of medicine has made it colder and more detached.

Dr. Robin Watson, radiology-department chairman at Memorial Sloan-Kettering Cancer Center [in New York], says: "The doctor-patient relationship has been lost in the hurly-burly of medical advances, but correct treatment or an early diagnosis may be better for you than holding your hand."

All aspects of medical care have been affected by technology. However, it is perhaps most visible in four major areas—heart disease, cancer, kidney failure and newborn infants.

Heart Disease

Every year, roughly sixty thousand Americans undergo coronary bypass surgery, the most common heart operation in the United States.

The patient wakes up in the intensive-care unit—the ICU. An intra-aorta balloon has been inserted to help the heart pump blood. A respirator does the breathing. A kidney-dialysis machine takes over in case of kidney failure. Standing by is defibrillation equipment, whose strong electrical currents restore the normal heartbeat.

An automated blood-gas analyzer measures how much oxygen is getting to other organs, a key indication of how well the patient is doing. According to the National Heart, Lung and Blood Institute, improvements in monitoring patients have cut down deaths in hospitals by almost a third in the last ten years. At the center of the ICU is the display panel. All the heartbeats in the ward are green dots bouncing across the television screen, and they are watched continuously by a technician. In the ICU, the machines monitor the patients, and the people monitor the machines.

Technology, however, begins long before the heart patient gets into the intensive- or coronary-care unit.

Just to diagnose certain conditions may take a machine, a computer and a technician, and a specialist to interpret the results. In the last five years, echocardiography, using ultrasound, has become an important tool. A scanning device little larger than a fist arcs back and forth across the chest. Sound waves are bounced off the soft tissues of the heart, mapping the cardiovascular landscape.

In the next room, a TV screen displays the computerized picture. Dr. Donald King of Columbia Presbyterian Medical Center in New York says: "The use of ultrasound is an incredible boon to cardiology. It means we can detect silent abnormalities we could never detect before."

Even so, Dr. Nicholas J. Fortuin, assistant professor of cardiovascular medicine at Johns Hopkins, demurs: "For every 2 people in the ICU, there are 10 million people with heart disease who don't need echocardiography or heart surgery. All too often a test substitutes for a doctor who isn't asking enough questions."

Machines themselves are not infallible. During an electrical brownout, cardiac monitors at one major hospital indicated that a patient's heart had stopped pumping blood. The treatment for this is swift and drastic—strong drugs or countershock therapy. In reality, the patient was fine. The low voltage in the power supply had introduced this problem on the display panel. But the physician looking only at the panel was about to start treatment.

Cancer

Technology dominates the treatment of cancer, beginning with the diagnosis. The patient lies on a stretcher inside a machine that hits the body with X-rays from many different angles as a ring of instruments rotates back and forth. The X-ray images are fed into a computer, which then reconstructs a three-dimensional picture on the TV screen.

To the health community, the arrival in recent years of this technique—called computerized axial tomography (CAT)—marks a revolution in diagnostic procedures.

Unlike previous methods such as the Potts Concentric Chair, which injects air into the spine and then turns the patient upside down, the CAT scanner is painless and relatively safe. It can also be used on outpatients.

In addition to detecting tumors, the body scanner tells the radiologist where to shoot his beams, the surgeon exactly where to operate and the pharmacologist about the effectiveness of drug therapy. For instance—

A fifteen-year-old girl is being treated for osteogenic sarcoma, or cancer of the leg. The body scan monitors how well chemotherapy is shrinking the tumor. Another diagnostic technique, the angiogram, outlines the major blood vessel in the leg. When the tumor has shrunk and is not touching the blood vessel, the surgeon can attempt a radical procedure: Cut the leg open from the hip to the ankle, take out the bone, replace it with an artifical one and hook the blood vessel up again. Without these techniques to pinpoint the tumor and the blood vessel, such an operation couldn't be done and the whole leg would be amputated.

Particle Bombardment. In the radiation center are big and advanced machines such as the linear accelerator, which bombards the patient with particles.

Physicists use computers to plot the dose and the path of these particles to the tumor much as planning the trajectory of a spacecraft to the moon. Purpose: to kill the malignant cells without destroying the surrounding normal cells—and the allowable error is small. A difference of 5 to 10 percent in the radiation dosage can seriously affect the outcome.

At present, there is rising interest in high-energy particles that penetrate deep inside the body. Whole-body scanning for patients with Hodgkin's disease, for example, has produced good results as the X-ray beams reach otherwise-inaccessible lymph nodes throughout the body.

Under way is research with charged particles, which explode at the end of their path, to see if they could be aimed in such a way that they would burst within the tumor and spare the rest of the body. Another approach is to implant radioactive seeds within the tumor.

While radiation treatments alone are used for some cancers, the trend now is toward a combination approach using surgery, radiation and drugs. Even so, the major malignancies such as lung and breast cancer still elude the best and most expensive tools of medical science.

Not for the lack of trying: Patients undergo long and painful therapies to stay alive. But one of the disadvantages of radiation therapy—and therapy with drugs or surgery—is that they lower a person's immunological system, making him more vulnerable to diseases.

In hospitals across the country, the radiation machines and banks of computers illustrate what Dr. Lewis Thomas, president of Memorial Sloane-Kettering, calls "halfway technology"—expensive, relatively ineffective and often risky and painful procedures used to diagnose and treat diseases which medical science does not yet understand. Dr. Thomas makes this point:

When polio still baffled physicians, treatments such as the iron lung were expensive, painful and relatively ineffective. Once medical science unlocks the cause of a disease, effective technology such as the vaccine for polio is usually cheap and effective. For cancer, however—

"The cost is at its highest and the technology at its most complex, when we are only halfway along," say Dr. Thomas.

Kidney Disease

A success story is unfolding from technology's impact on kidney disease.

Over thirty thousand Americans are alive today because of dialysis machines that take over the kidney's blood-purifying function. More transplants are being successfully performed; three-month-old babies have received new kidneys. Young women with transplanted kidneys have even borne children.

Only in the last few years, with technology's aid, have researchers known how to recognize telltale genetic differences of white blood cells, which will determine whether or not the body will accept the foreign organ. Individual genetic characteristics are fed into a giant computer that then matches recipients with donors. Last February [1977], a kidney from a Russian teen-ager killed in a Moscow traffic accident was matched with a thirty-two-year-old former construction worker in New York.

The kidney itself is preserved for up to seventy-two hours in a machine filled with nutrient fluids to substitute for a live body. Research is under way to preserve the organ longer, a step toward creating a national kidney bank.

From a technological point of view, the actual operation is the simplest part of the process. In contrast, the recovery period is critical: Will the transplanted kidney "take"? Complex blood tests are performed to detect signs of rejection and an X-ray scan three times a week determines how well the new kidney is functioning.

After the patient leaves the hospital, the monitoring continues. At the two-year mark, the chances that a transplanted kidney is still successful are 50-50.

The costs of treating kidney failure are as spectacular as the technology. Kidney dialysis in a hospital reaches $26,000 a year for each person. The combined costs for transplants and kidney dialysis is $600 million for Medicare patients alone. "In the past, technology only dealt with acute episodic illness," explains Dr. Samuel Kountz of the Downstate Medical Center in Brooklyn, New York, who has done over five hundred transplants. "Now we're talking about chronic disease. It's a never-ending treatment, and the costs can only go up."

Newborn Infants

More than ever before, the outlook for premature babies is optimistic. The National Foundation/March of Dimes says that 80,000 "premies" are born every year and 73 percent survive.

A newborn premie is quickly placed in the isolette, a plastic-encased crib to protect him from cold and infection. An automatic warmer keeps his environment at 75 degrees; a motorized humidifier keeps air circulating. Four portholes let nurses reach in and touch the infant.

Usually babies born six weeks early have troubled breathing. A trachea tube is put down the infant's throat and attached to a ventilator. In the place of the umbilical cord, tubes are inserted to administer fluids, monitor blood pressure and draw out blood for tests.

The critical question is how much oxygen to give the

premature baby. Too much can result in blindness and permanent lung damage. Too little ends in brain damage or death. Improvements in monitoring oxygen levels over the last five years have greatly reduced these problems.

But several studies have shown that the incidence of lingering abnormalities is higher among premies. It is estimated that one such infant in five will have some defect.

More troubling are babies born with severe disorders that can now be cured by modern medical techniques.

Five years ago, for instance, babies born with "short-gut syndrome" never survived. Now surgery can reconstruct their intestines so they will be able to absorb food. But both mental and motor development are delayed. At one hospital, a ten-month-old baby thus treated has never been out of the special unit, is half his normal size and cannot speak.

Perhaps the *Wunderkind* of medical technology is the seven-year-old boy from Houston who has never left the plastic bubble that has been his home since birth. Because he suffers from a rare deficiency in immunity, he cannot fight off the common viruses and bacteria. So far the boy is healthy both emotionally and physically. But his future is uncertain until technology can enable him to enter the real world.

Is it all worthwhile? Says Kathy White, in charge of the special neonatal unit at Johns Hopkins: "You can't *not* take advantage of the medical technology we now have if there is a chance."

III. THE QUESTION OF PAYMENT

EDITOR'S INTRODUCTION

Who foots the bill for medical care in America? Ultimately, the consumer—out of his or her pocket, or through insurance premiums and taxes.

The first selection in this section, taken from the *Public Interest* and written by Martin Feldstein, an economist with a special interest in medical-care costs, examines the impact of insurance itself on hospital costs. In the second selection, from *Current History*, Dorothy P. Rice, director of the National Center for Health Statistics, takes stock of this mixed system of financing.

There follows a New York *Times* article by John P. Allegrante, a health-care specialist, telling what a catastrophic illness cost his father—in money. Like millions of self-employed Americans, the senior Allegrante could not afford private health insurance, yet he was considered too well off to qualify for public assistance.

The public role in financing the medical-care system has grown in the past decade. Medicaid, a federal and state program, and Medicare, a federal program, are largely responsible for that growth. A brief excerpt from a *Current History* article points up the inadequacies of the Medicaid program and the built-in causes of them.

The next contributions to this section examine the abuse of Medicaid by a small minority of profiteers, the inevitable attempt by states to check Medicaid costs, and the resulting retrenchments.

Medicaid and Medicare are beset with inefficiencies, but by most accounts they are accomplishing what they set out to do—provide medical care to those who can least afford it. As with many successful programs, however, new problems have been created even while old ones are being solved.

HOSPITAL COSTS AND INSURANCE [1]

The explosion of hospital costs is now the central problem of our national health-care policy. Congress and the Administration are actively considering plans to impose direct controls on the costs of more than seven thousand individual hospitals. More generally, now that Medicare and Medicaid provide benefits for the aged and the poor, it is the rapid increase of hospital costs that provides the primary impetus for national health insurance. Unfortunately, the current policy initiatives generally reflect a misunderstanding of why hospital costs have risen so rapidly and of how hospital-cost inflation is very different than the other types of inflation that trouble our economy.

The magnitude of the increase in hospital costs has been overwhelmingly greater than the general rise in prices. From 1950 to 1976, the overall consumer price index (which measures the cost of all goods and services bought by consumers) rose about 125 percent. During the same period, medical-care costs as a whole rose nearly twice as much, 240 percent. But the upsurge in the cost of hospital care was much more dramatic. Average cost per patient-day was only $16 in 1950. By 1976, it was about $175, an increase of more than 1,000 percent.

While everyone is aware that hospital costs have risen rapidly, there is little understanding of why this has happened at such an unprecedented rate. Much has been written about the rise in hospital wage-rates and the supposedly low rate of increase in productivity among hospital staff. But such "explanations" miss the real nature of the problem. For there are two—and really only two—key ingredients to understanding the rise in hospital costs: *the changing nature of the hospital product,* and *the impact of insurance.* Of these, the second is the more crucial—and largely explains the first.

[1] From "The High Cost of Hospitals and What to Do About It," by Martin Feldstein, author, educator, Harvard professor, president of National Bureau of Economic Research. *Public Interest.* 48:40–5. Summer '77. Copyright 1977 by National Affairs, Inc. Reprinted by permission.

The Changing Hospital Product

The most obvious thing about hospital care today is that it is very different from what it was twenty-five years ago. Today's care is more complex, more sophisticated, and, it is to be hoped, more effective.

The rapid rise in hospital costs unquestionably reflects this rapidly changing product. The rate of hospital-cost inflation, therefore, cannot be compared without qualification to the rate of inflation of most other goods in the consumer price index. The consumer price index tries to measure the cost of buying an *unchanged* bundle of goods and services. But the meaning of cost inflation in hospital care is not that consumers are paying much more for the same old product, but that they are buying a different and much more expensive product today. Hospital-cost inflation is therefore quite different from the other types of inflation in our economy. To understand the nature of this problem, we must ask why hospital care has become much more sophisticated—and therefore much more expensive.

Higher incomes and greater education have undoubtedly played some role in increasing the demand for sophisticated hospital care, and scientific discoveries have obviously changed the technological possibilities in hospitals. *But the major reason, I believe, for hospital-cost inflation has been the very rapid growth in insurance.*

In addition to providing protection against unforeseen medical expenses, health insurance substantially lowers the net price of care that the patient pays out-of-pocket at the time he consumes services. There is now substantial evidence that patients, guided by their doctors, demand more services and more expensive services when a large part of the cost is offset by insurance.

Some simple but striking numbers will illustrate this point. In 1950, when average cost per patient-day was a little less than $16, private insurance and government programs paid 49 percent of hospital bills. This meant that, on the average, the net cost to a patient of a day of care was just under $8. By 1975, average cost per patient-day had jumped to about $152—but private and public insurance were paying 88 percent of the hospital bill, leaving a net cost to the patient of only $18. Thus, although the cost of providing a day of hospital care had increased more than ninefold (from $16 to $152), the *net* cost to patients had only just about doubled (from $8 to $18). Moreover, the general increase in the prices of all goods and services meant that $18 in 1975 could only buy as much as $8 in 1950! So in *real* terms, the net cost to the patient at the time of illness has not changed at all during the past twenty-five years.

Even if we disregard Medicare, Medicaid, and other government programs, the picture is not very different. In 1950, private insurance paid 37 percent of private hospital bills. That meant that, on average, the net cost to a private patient for a day of hospital care was just under $10. By 1975 private insurance was paying for 79 percent of privately financed hospital care. The average net cost to the patient at the time of illness, therefore, was only $32 per day—not the $152 incurred by the hospital. In the prices of 1950, this $32 is equivalent to $14. In *real* terms, the net cost per day to the patient had only increased by $4.

Looked at somewhat differently, with 79 percent of private hospital bills now paid by insurance, an extra $10 of expensive care costs the patient only $2 out-of-pocket. It is not surprising, therefore, that patients and their doctors continue to encourage the growing sophistication (and expense) of hospital care.

I think this is the essence of the hospital-cost inflation problem: *Increased insurance has induced hospitals to improve their product and provide much more expensive and sophisticated care.*

The Usual Explanations

Before considering the implications of this explanation, let me contrast it with the usual reasons offered for the rise in hospital costs. These traditionally boil down to four ideas: (1) Hospitals are inefficient; (2) labor costs have risen particularly rapidly; (3) hospitals have had a low rise in technical progress; and (4) hospital supply has not kept up with increasing demand. Each of these notions is basically incorrect.

Perhaps the most frequently heard explanation of rising hospital costs is that hospitals are technologically and managerially inefficient. But even if there are good reasons for criticizing the efficiency of hospitals, there is absolutely no reason to believe their inefficiency has been rapidly increasing over the past two decades. Inefficiency cannot possibly account for a 1,000-percent increase in hospital costs! It cannot begin to account for a significant fraction of that overwhelming increase.

Rising labor costs are also frequently cited as the primary cause of hospital-cost inflation. It is true that wages and salaries constitute a large share of hospital costs, and that hospital wages have risen more rapidly than wages in the general economy. Nevertheless, this does not begin to account for the rise in hospital costs. From 1955 to 1975, labor-cost per patient-day rose at a rate of 9 percent a year. But *as a fraction of the total hospital bill, labor costs actually decreased from 62 percent in 1955 to 53 percent in 1975.* In other words, nonlabor costs rose faster than labor costs. Moreover, about one third of the increase in labor costs was due to a rise in the number of personnel per patient-day rather than an increase in hospital wage rates. I recently calculated that the earnings of hospital employees rose at 6.3 percent a year from 1955 to 1975, while the average earnings of all private nonfarm workers rose at 4.5 percent. If the rate of increase of hospital wages had been held to this 4.5-percent national average, the overall rise in the average cost of a day of hospital care would have been reduced from 9.9 percent a year to 8.8 percent. In other words, *the rise of hospital wages in excess of the national average rate of wage increase can only account for about one tenth of the high rate of hospital-cost inflation.*

The third common explanation is that hospital-cost inflation is the result of a low rate of technical progress. I think this is clearly and obviously false. Hospitals have been the scene of extremely rapid technical changes. But these changes differ from those in other industries: They have not been cost-reducing. Technological progress in hospitals does not involve making the old product more cheaply, but making a new range of products that are more expensive.

Why have hospitals moved toward increasingly expensive ways of doing more things for patients, rather than toward providing old services more cheaply? Although some of this merely reflects the path of scientific progress, I believe it can be shown that it is our method of financing health services that primarily determines the pattern of technological change itself. Hospitals would not be buying the latest, expensive medical technology if they could not afford it. What permits them to afford it is our mode of insuring against hospital costs.

The final traditional explanation is that hospital costs have risen because supply has not kept up with demand. Usually, economic analysis of ordinary markets emphasizes that prices rise because supply does not increase as rapidly as demand. But in the case of hospitals, I think the opposite is true. *It is precisely because supply has kept pace with demand that hospital costs have gone up.* Hospitals have responded to the increased demand and increased willingness to pay for sophisticated services by providing them, and costs have gone up accordingly. The increase in demand has induced a rapid rise in the supply of a *more expensive* type of hospital care.

This brings me back to my original contention that the rise in hospital costs reflects a change in the product, largely induced by the growth of insurance. But this explanation of the rise in hospital costs raises an awkward question. Implicit in every discussion of hospital-cost inflation is the assumption that the rise in cost has been excessive and should not be allowed to continue at the same rate in the future. But if this rise reflects a change in product rather than an increase in inefficiency or a low rate of technological progress, why is it really a problem?

The answer in brief is that the current type of costly medical care does not really correspond to what consumers or their physicians would regard as appropriate if their choices were not distorted by insurance. The effect of prepaying health care through insurance, both private and public, is to encourage hospitals to provide a more expensive product than the consumers actually wish to pay for. And in the end, we do pay for it—in ever higher insurance premiums.

Although the consumer eventually pays the full cost of the expensive care through higher insurance premiums, *at the time of illness* the choice of the patient and his physician reflects the *net* out-of-pocket cost of the care. Because this net out-of-pocket cost appears so modest, the patient and physician choose to buy more expensive care than they would if the patient were not so well insured. In this way, our current method of financing hospital care denies patients and their physicians the opportunity to choose effectively between higher-cost and lower-cost hospital care.

Why Patients Overinsure

If insurance is responsible for such an inappropriate expansion in the demand for expensive care, why has insurance grown so rapidly? In part, this growth reflects a family's rational demand for protection against unexpected illness. It is unfortunate but inevitable that this process tends to be self-perpetuating. *The high cost of care induces families to buy more complete insurance, and the growth of insurance induces the hospital to produce more expensive care.*

But this demand for protection cannot explain the comprehensive "first-dollar insurance"—i.e., insurance for all costs up to a specified limit—that now exists. Current insurance is often inadequate in protecting the family against the substantial bills that can cause real hardship. Why have Americans bought such complete coverage for relatively small bills? Why have they been willing to pay for insurance that provides little real protection against catastrophic illness but induces them to buy more expensive and sophisticated care for less serious illnesses?

Most insurance is now group insurance and, more specifically, insurance bought for employee groups. Decisions on the scope of coverage and on coinsurance rates and deductibles are generally made in collective bargaining by expert representatives of labor and management. Why would such experts forgo higher wages in order to obtain excessive, shallow insurance? *The answer, I believe, lies in the tax treatment of premiums.*

Government policies encourage insurance by a tax deduction and exclusion that now cost the Treasury more than $6 billion a year. Individuals can deduct about half of the premiums they pay for health insurance. More important, employer payments for insurance are excluded from the taxable income of the employee as well as the employer. These premiums are also not subject to Social Security taxes or state income taxes.

Thus, even for a relatively low-income family, the inducement to buy insurance can be quite substantial. Because of the income and payroll taxes, a married man who has two children and earns $8,000 a year will take home an additional $70 for each $100 the employer adds to his income. If the employer buys health insurance instead, the full $100 can be applied against the premium and there is no tax to be paid. In this case, the dollar buys nearly 50 percent more in health-care services if paid through an insurance premium than if paid in wages to individuals who then buy the care directly. For workers in high tax brackets, the incentive is stronger.

I believe the subsidy is strong enough to induce employees and unions to choose higher insurance instead of higher wages. The primary effect of this insurance is to distort the pattern of medical care and to exacerbate the rising cost of hospital care. Moreover, this subsidy, which costs taxpayers several billion dollars a year, is quite regressive: The subsidy is greatest for middle- and upper-income employees in high-wage industries. In short, the current tax treatment of insurance premiums, particularly the exclusion of employer payments from the employees' taxable incomes, is a costly, regressive, and inefficient aspect of our tax system.

PUBLIC AND PRIVATE FINANCING [2]

In 1965, the year before implementation of the Medi-care and Medicaid programs, medical care expenditures totaled $38.9 billion, 5.9 percent of the GNP [Gross National Product]; in 1970, they totaled $69.2 billion, 7.2 percent. The $139.3 billion expended in 1976 represented 8.6 percent of the GNP.

Hospital care is the largest single item in health expenditures; it amounted to $55.4 billion in fiscal year 1976, nearly 40 percent of the total health outlay. In 1965, hospital care represented about one third of the total outlay. The rise in hospital expenditures has been caused by increased costs of labor and supplies, increased demand (with the growth of private health insurance and government programs), and costly technological changes.

Nursing-home care is the most rapidly growing component of medical care, with expenditures increasing from $3.8 billion (6 percent of the total outlay) in 1970 to $10.6 billion (or 8 percent of the total) in 1976. This component will continue to grow as the number of elderly persons in the population increases.

Among other components of personal health-care expenditures, physicians' services cost $26.3 billion in 1976 (19 percent of the total outlay); dentist services, $8.6 billion (6 percent); and drugs and drug sundries, $11.2 billion (8 percent). Expenditures for construction of hospitals, nursing homes, medical clinics, and medical research facilities

[2] From "Health Facilities in the United States," by Dorothy P. Rice, director, National Center for Health Statistics, U.S. Department of Health, Education, and Welfare. *Current History*. 72:211–12. My./Je. '77. Copyright © 1977 by Current History, Inc. Reprinted by permission.

accounted for $5.0 billion and medical research for $3.3 billion.

As medical care expenditures have increased, the source of financing has changed dramatically. Public programs, primarily Medicare and Medicaid, have taken over more and more of the burden of paying for hospital care. In fiscal 1966, the year before Medicare, the private sector, including private health insurance, contributed 64 percent of the $14.2 billion total; the federal government paid 13 percent, and state and local governments spent the remaining 23 percent. In fiscal 1976, the portion of hospital expenditures paid by the private sector declined to about 45 percent. Together, government and private health insurance paid over 90 percent of hospital expenses in 1976, with government paying 55 percent and private insurance 35 percent.

The financing of nursing-home care has also changed significantly as the result of Medicare and Medicaid. Both these programs support care for eligible persons in skilled nursing facilities; Medicaid also provides coverage in intermediate level facilities for persons who need long-term care but do not require the degree of care available in skilled nursing facilities. In 1976, the government paid over half the costs of nursing-home care, chiefly through federal funds, in comparison with 43 percent in fiscal year 1966. Most of the remaining cost is paid by individuals and their families.

Private funds continue to pay most of the bill for physicians' services, but the public share increased from 7 percent in fiscal 1965 to 25 percent in 1976. Consumers paid 39 percent directly in 1976; health insurance paid 36 percent. For dental expenses and the costs of drugs and sundries, consumers continue to pay more than 80 percent of the costs.

The growth of private health insurance and public programs have greatly reduced the consumer's direct share of the costs of health care, notably hospital care.

UNINSURED IN AMERICA [3]

... [In the spring of 1977] my father survived a heart attack. Now that he is recovering, we are not so much concerned about his physical condition as we are about his financial situation. While he has survived the heart attack, he may not survive the bills.

My father is among the estimated hundreds of thousands of Americans who have no health insurance. I have had to repeat this fact to incredulous hospital administrators and his physicians. And I have been made to feel that my father has broken some unwritten law.

He spent eight days in a coronary-care unit at a cost of $220 per day and another two weeks in a semiprivate hospital room at approximately $100 per day. If my arithmetic is correct, he can expect a hospital bill of about $3,160. This, of course, does not include diagnostic costs or his cardiologist's fee. I figure that a conservative estimate of my father's medical expenses should total about $5,000. And he may still need an operation!

To some people that amount may not seem like much money. But to a fifty-eight-year-old man who is a self-employed barber in rural Dutchess County, New York, that amount is enough to make one worry; I see the worry in my father's face. Self-employed barbers in rural Dutchess County don't make that much money. My father hasn't paid income tax in years now (since the long-haired Beatles came to America).

To be sure, my father is a small man, both literally and figuratively. Although he has never made a great deal of money in his barbershop, he did at least make enough money to, as the saying goes, "make ends meet." He has always been able to pay most of his bills and taxes on time. In short, my father and mother have been good citizens,

[3] Article entitled "Well, Who Needs Life Savings?" by John P. Allegrante, specialist in health and safety education. New York *Times*. p 23. Ap. 27, '77. © 1977 by The New York Times Company. Reprinted by permission.

honest, hard-working, and have in their own small way contributed to the economic good of our country. However, he is now likely to be ruined financially by medical bills.

What about our system of Social Security and welfare that purports to help those in need and into which my father has paid dutifully all of his working life, you ask? Will Medicaid not pay for his medical expenses? My answer is that we have filed for medical assistance, but that is no guarantee that he will receive Medicaid. Even if he does, the Catch-22 clause will be that what pitifully little financial assets he does have left will now be a liability, and he will, in effect, be responsible for paying a rather large deductible.

My father—like a good number of other self-employed, working-class Americans—falls into an unhappy category of many thousands who can neither afford the escalating costs of the monthly private health insurance premiums, nor meet the required means test of Medicaid. Financially, my father and others like him find themselves in the unenviable situation of being in a "no-man's land" when it comes to affording adequate health-care for their families.

The question that arises, of course, is how can this be? Should it be in a society that values universal education and a voice in free government as inalienable human rights that health care not be considered the same? Why must health care continue to have financial barriers?

It is my business as an academic to be familiar with the issues that confront this country in delivering and financing health care and, moreover, to educate people to understand government policies and to help change these policies if change is warranted. Yet, it has not been until now that even I realized the urgency of the situation that faces literally hundreds of thousands of Americans who have either no health insurance or coverage that is inadequate.

The present "system" of delivering and financing health care simply fails to be egalitarian and pluralistic, despite the high-sounding claims of some politicians.

The much-needed legislation that would help to finance

health care for *all* Americans is long overdue. Health care and its costs are now too large a problem for too large a number of Americans to be ignored. Ask my father if you don't believe me.

MEDICAID PROGRAMS [4]

Medicaid is a federal/state program. Each state administers its own Medicaid program and determines its own eligibility requirements and benefit package, although the federal government has established minimum requirements. The federal share is based on a complicated formula, involving per capita income in the state. In effect, Medicaid is tied to the "welfare" system; it is run like a welfare program and has inherited all the problems associated with the welfare system.

Inequities abound in Medicaid. Because the federal contribution depends on the size of the state's program and because larger, wealthier states have better programs, they tend to receive larger dollar contributions from the federal government. Because the states have such leeway, wide variation in benefit levels occur from state to state. For example, in 1972, average medical payments ranged from $50 in Mississippi to $1,150 in New York. Three states—New York, Massachusetts, and California—spend 50 percent of all Medicaid funds. The poorest, most rural states have the most inadequate programs.

When the Medicaid program was established, estimates of its growth were modest. The reality has far exceeded expectations. . . . The sixfold increase in Medicaid expenditures has been a major source of dissatisfaction. The governors, for example, are now claiming that Medicaid is their number one financing problem; they allege that it is forcing them to bankruptcy. According to a report from the National Governor's Conference:

[4] From "Federal Involvement in Health Care After 1945," by Leda R. Judd, former director of national affairs for the National Urban Coalition. *Current History*. 72:206, 227. My./Je. '77. Copyright © 1977 by Current History, Inc. Reprinted by permission.

Medicaid has become the most rapidly escalating cost of state budgets. From a modest beginning of $250 million a decade ago the program's annual cost has grown to $18 billion. By 1980 it's expected to surpass $30 billion, more than the entire national budget of most countries.

Because of these unmanageable costs, the governors are trying to cut back on the programs despite the hardships this will mean to many persons.

As with Medicare, health professionals have benefited greatly from Medicaid. In fact, Medicare and Medicaid have benefited the providers as much as the aged and needy. Charges that individual practitioners have received large sums of money from Medicaid and reports of other forms of fraud and abuse have led Congress to seek reform of the program. While reform is high on the legislative agenda, any major substantive changes are unlikely. Instead, some form of national health insurance will probably take over this program. Efforts to control costs will continue, however, and HEW [Department of Health, Education, and Welfare] has appointed its first Inspector General, who will have the responsibility for policing alleged Medicaid irregularities.

Other changes are also coming. Under the recent HEW reorganization plan, both Medicare and Medicaid will be placed in a new HEW division, the Health Care Financing Administration, which "will provide basic quality control and will tackle strenuously the problems of fraud and abuse that so severely undermine our governmental health programs."

Despite its problems, Medicaid has not been an entirely negative experience. During 1976, it provided medical services for more than two million Americans—one out of every ten—including people who would not have been able to obtain care without the program. Low-income families now visit physicians more often than the well-to-do, and there is some evidence that mortality rates for low-income families are declining. For many poor children, the program has been particularly effective by focusing on the detection and treatment of childhood disease.

MEDICAID ABUSE [5]

"Our patients understand, all right, but we've had to go out of our way to convince our colleagues that we still practice medicine that is as good as you'll find anywhere in the country," Dr. William Hewlett said with quiet firmness. "We are not a 'mill'."

. . . Such remarks would [once] have seemed curiously combative coming from a soft-spoken, fifty-six-year-old pediatrician. But a Senate committee report issued last week alleging widespread mismanagement and fraud in the nationwide $15-billion-a-year federal- and state-funded Medicaid program for the poor has prompted extraordinary reactions from many quarters here.

Some individuals and groups have responded defensively while others have snapped back with bitterness and even disdain at the probe, which included reports of healthy people being diagnosed as sick in New York City "Medicare mills." Still others, professionals like Dr. Hewlett and his associates at the Carter Community Health Center, have remained low-key, convinced that the accusations have unfairly tainted the innocent as well as the guilty.

It is a situation that no one at the center—located in the world-weary heart of south Jamaica, a low-income, predominantly black and Hispanic neighborhood in Queens—wants to think about, and yet it is one that none of them can escape.

Created in the late 1960s by thirty-two black doctors, dentists, biochemists and pharmacists, each of whom invested several thousand dollars to cover the two mortgages on the $700,000 construction cost, the one-story facility was designed as a high-quality alternative to existing health centers.

"When Medicaid first came out in 1967, there were store-

[5] Article entitled "N.Y. Doctors Fight 'Medicaid Mill' Tag," by David C. Berliner, staff correspondent. Washington *Post*. p A 8. S. 7, '76. Copyright © 1976, Field Enterprises Inc., reproduced through the courtesy of Field Newspaper Syndicate.

fronts popping up all over our area," Hewlett said during an informal tour through the clean, brightly lit, uncrowded building. "Patients were getting very inferior care, and we got reports that there were wires strung from wall to wall with sheets draped across them to form examining rooms.

"When we checked, we found that there were no facilities for the physicians to wash their hands and that they were moving from chair to chair extracting teeth or doing whatever. It was absolutely terrible. That's when we got together here."

Unlike all but a half dozen other so-called "free-standing" facilities and like most, if not all, of the hospitals in the city, the Carter Center was granted Article 28 status by the state. The classification brought along with it certain financial benefits, such as a guaranteed $32.43-per-visit fee paid by Medicaid, but also the kind of strict regulation by municipal and state agencies not placed on non-"A-28" facilities.

"Nowadays, when you say Medicaid center, most people don't know there's a difference," said Dr. Shelton Aiken, a tall, stocky, forty-seven-year-old dentist who doubles as the Carter Center's board chairman. "The investigation of these places is necessary—no two ways about it—but we are being lumped into that group when we shouldn't be."

According to records provided by Aiken, the center last year [1975] treated 59,609 patients at its main building and at a smaller annex four miles away. Of those, 42,289 (or 71 percent) were covered by Medicaid, while the rest paid directly for their treatment. Total billings amounted to $1.7 million, with $1.4 million of that assessed to Medicaid.

Fees—one of the major issues in the current investigation—were, and continue to be, based on set scales.

"Except for six of our members, we all have private practices," said Hewlett, who said he derives two thirds of his income from his salary paid by the center. "We charge the same fee to private patients whether they see us in our personal offices or at the center. An initial visit to me would cost $25, and each followup would be $12, plus the cost of any inoculations that might be required.

"For Medicaid patients we receive $32.43 per visit per patient, regardless of how little or how much is done. However, while that may seem like a lot, especially when the visit is only for a quick, relatively inexpensive treatment or examination, it balances out."

In support of that argument, Dr. John W. V. Cordice, a surgeon-partner, said he had performed an operation earlier in the day to repair an umbilical hernia. "If that was a private patient, the charges would amount to $350 or $400," he said. "As it is, we'll be lucky if we get back $40 from Medicaid . . . when we get it back."

"In fact," Hewlett said, "in the past few years we have even tried to get a higher per capita rate, but have been turned down each time. They've even lowered it. Not that we are in any financial difficulties, but the truth is, we're just about making it here. We're just trying to keep our heads above water."

Cordice said, "Hospitals—whether through political power or whatever—charge incredible fees for patients who come for treatment in their emergency rooms. Then the hospital gets $80, $90, $100 or even more back from the government. This has gotten so expensive that it has become untenable. There is no reason why Medicaid should support open-heart projects, kidney machines and other special programs. Right now the hospitals are defraying their costs through Medicaid."

On the other hand, Aiken contends, exceptionally low fees paid to private practitioners "lead to trouble."

"In an average office," he said, "a tooth extraction costs $15 to $20, although Medicaid only pays somewhere between $4 and $7. So this man has got to see a lot of people to make up that difference, and that's why they become hustlers rather than practitioners. Their thing gets to be strictly volume."

"Something has got to be done," Aiken concluded with

a shrug of his shoulders, "and it has got to be done very, very soon. If the government doesn't straighten out the paperwork, adjust the fees and send more inspectors into the field, this program won't mean a thing. The losers are not going to be the doctors, but the very patients everyone is trying to help."

MEDICAID RETRENCHMENT [6]

Medicaid, the ten-year-old federal-state partnership for providing the poor with medical care, seems headed into a period of retrenchment because of rising medical costs and mounting budgetary difficulties in many states.

According to officials at the Department of Health, Education, and Welfare (HEW), eighteen states recently initiated programs for cutting back Medicaid services. And several other states and the District of Columbia currently are considering Medicaid-cutback proposals.

Few of the cutback programs or proposals would diminish the number of persons eligible for medical assistance under Medicaid, but the retrenchment means that the recipients will begin getting less out of the programs. The basic program will remain intact, but the "optionals" are being pared.

Inflation Plus Recession

About 22.5 million Americans now receive Medicaid benefits, at a cost of $13 billion. The Federal Government pays most of this; the states pay from 22 to 50 percent, depending on per-capita income. The states administer their own programs.

But states are finding it increasingly difficult to maintain current services on available funds. "It's part of a general tightening up," says David Smith, commissioner of Maine's Department of Human Services, which has just slashed about $2 million from the $14.4-million state Medicaid

[6] From article by Robert W. Merry, staff writer. *National Observer*. p 5. Ja. 17, '76. Reprinted with permission of The National Observer. © Dow Jones & Company, Inc. 1976. All Rights Reserved.

budget. Adds an HEW spokesman: "Medical care prices have increased at a much higher rate than general inflation, and with the recession the states aren't collecting as much in taxes. So Medicaid is susceptible to cutbacks; it's sort of open-ended and can be pared with a very fine knife."

An example of the soaring costs is the Washington, D.C., Medicaid budget. In 1970 it was $16.3 million; in 1975, $94 million. Enrolment is up to 182,256 from 109,000 in 1970. And the average cost of services per person shot up to $629 annually from $178 in 1970.

"It is easy to see why our department is talking about cost containment in the Medicaid program," says a spokesman for the city's Department of Human Resources.

Cost-containment efforts, in Washington and elsewhere, mean that many persons on Medicaid will be paying more for such things as prescription drugs, dental care, and "prosthetic devices" such as eyeglasses, hearing aids, and artificial limbs. In addition, some states have constricted certain mandatory services—the length of a patient's hospital stay that will be covered, for example, or the number of doctor visits he may make in a year.

Mandatory Services

The program's mandatory services are inpatient and outpatient hospital care, lab services, family planning, physician service, nursing-home care and home-health services for persons over twenty-one, and early screening, diagnosis, and treatment programs for persons under twenty-one. Optional services include dental and mental-health care, payment for prescription drugs, services such as podiatry and chiropractic, and prosthetic devices.

But federal officials explain that the program doesn't stipulate how complete the coverage must be for mandatory services. As a result, many states are paring costs by reducing their coverage in these areas, thus increasing the cost to patients who want the service. In addition, states are eliminating, or adding small costs for, the optional services.

An example of cost cutbacks is a recent New Jersey

program that: requires Medicaid recipients to pay 25 cents for each prescription; eliminates reimbursements for certain drugs; reduces slightly the state's fees to pharmacies for handling Medicaid accounts; reduces by 10 percent reimbursement rates for many health services; reduces by 40 percent reimbursements for laboratory services; and reduces coverage for services such as replacement of eyeglasses and dentures.

The saving from these measures, according to government figures: $23 million from a New Jersey operating Medicaid budget of about $400 million.

MEDICARE [7]

Medicare, the largest of the federal health financing programs, is a health insurance program in two parts: Part A, the hospital insurance program, and Part B, the supplementary medical insurance program. The hospital insurance program covers hospital, long-term and home health care and is financed by Social Security taxes. Part B covers physician fees, out-patient hospital services, and other selected services like physical therapy. It is financed through a monthly premium (currently around $7) paid by the enrollee and by general federal tax revenues. Over 95 percent of Americans aged sixty-five and older are covered by Part A and most of those persons also elect Part B. Medicare also requires that beneficiaries pay a "deductible" (the first $92 of their hospital bill) and "co-insurance" (a portion of each day's hospital bill after sixty days).

Medicare, of course, accounted for an increase in the utilization of health services by the elderly. After Medicare went into effect, the use of these services by persons over sixty-five increased more than 25 percent; and, as utilization increased, so did costs.

Both hospital charges and physician fees began to spiral

[7] From "Federal Involvement in Health Care After 1945," by Leda R. Judd, former director of national affairs, National Urban Coalition. *Current History*. 72:206. My./Je. '77. Copyright © 1977 by Current History, Inc. Reprinted by permission.

upward. The massive infusion of federal funds contributed to this growth for several reasons: doctors and hospitals no longer needed to provide any free or "charitable" care, because money was available to pay almost everyone's bills; more patients could afford to use more medical and hospital services, and did; and, most important, except when price controls were in effect under the economic stabilization program, doctors could raise fees with impunity, because Medicare payments to providers were based on the "customary" fees charged by physicians in a given location.

Despite these problems, Medicare has undoubtedly improved the quality of care received and has enlarged access to care. A variety of federal standards for participating providers have been established. These standards range from record-keeping provisions to a review of the utilization patterns of the facility. They have upgraded the quality of care, particularly in smaller hospitals.

THE "RICH" MEDICARE DOCS [8]

During 1975 Dr. Charles D. Kelman, a New York City ophthalmologist, earned $412,757 for services paid by Medicare, the federal health-care program for the elderly.

Chesapeake Physicians of Baltimore received $844,294 in Medicare payments that year. And in Zumbrota, Minnesota (population 1,830), the Zumbrota Health Facility took in $22,293,171 from the government.

All these revelations, and more, can be found in a half-inch thick list published . . . [mid-March 1977] by the Department of Health, Education, and Welfare. The disclosure, produced to satisfy requests under the Freedom of Information Act, provided the names and addresses of physicians, clinics and group practices, and laboratories that earned $100,000 or more in Medicare services for 1975.

However well-intentioned, the federal disclosure contained enough errors and produced enough confusion to

[8] Article by Lawrence Mosher, staff writer. *National Observer.* p 2. Mr. 26, '77. Reprinted with permission of The National Observer. © Dow Jones & Company, Inc. 1977. All Rights Reserved.

make officials at the Social Security Administration wish
they had never heard of the law that led to publication of
the list.

"Guilt by Innuendo"

Social Security spokesmen reported that their Baltimore
office was ringing with angry doctors calling to complain.
One St. Louis doctor, they said, insisted he had been retired
for ten years. The American Medical Association criticized
the disclosures as establishing "guilt by innuendo"; the
AMA says the impression is created that doctors who receive large Medicare payments must somehow be doing
something illegal.

Take the examples used in this story. They are deceptive
unless fully explained, which often was not possible from
the information given in the list. The Zumbrota Health
Facility should have been listed as the Mayo Clinic, Rochester; Zumbrota is a town near Rochester. Chesapeake Physicians Professional Association numbers about two hundred doctors, all practicing at Baltimore's City Hospital.
Dr. Kelman employs a staff of two other ophthalmologists,
four technicians, and four secretaries. He reports that his
overhead costs exceed his Medicare payments. Such payments, he says, account for about 75 percent of his total
income.

A major cause of the confusion is the Social Security Administration's computerized billing system for Medicare.
Group practices and clinics are often listed under one doctor's name without giving the other names. Although the
Medicare list distinguished between "solo practitioners"
and "group/clinics," some newspapers and reporting services apparently did not make this clear.

A New List

What affronted some physicians, however, was the disclosure itself. "They made it sound like the doctors were
just pocketing the money," says Kelman. He received an
American Academy of Achievement award in 1969 for

developing an ultrasonic needle procedure for removing cataracts.

Kelman's surgical process, which he has taught to some 1,500 other ophthalmologists around the country, allows patients to go home the day after the operation. The standard operation requires an additional four days' hospitalization. Kelman figures he personally saves the government $240,000 a year in unnecessary hospitalization costs.

By week's end the Social Security Administration said it was preparing a new list that it hopes would eliminate the errors. The disclosures, however, appear to be a new aspect of Medicare operation that physicians will have to live with.

IV. THE QUESTION OF AVAILABILITY

EDITOR'S INTRODUCTION

New York City's Borough of Manhattan has 800 doctors for every 100,000 people; rural Mississippi has fewer than 50 for every 100,000. This pattern of imbalance is repeated throughout the nation. Inner-city areas are as poorly served as rural areas.

The results of this imbalance have been quantified: people who live in rural areas are twice as likely *never* to have had a physical examination as people who live in suburbia; and the chance that a black child will not be immunized against polio is one third higher than it is for a white child.

This section looks into the maldistribution of medical resources in the United States. It opens with an overview of the problem by Mary W. Herman, assistant professor of community health and preventive medicine at Jefferson Medical College in Philadelphia, in an article from *Current History* entitled "Meeting the Patient's Needs." Next, John B. Dunne, executive director of a New England health planning agency, explains why rural doctors are so few and discusses strategies that rural areas are using to lure physicians into service in their communities. The third selection, by Paul Starr, a Harvard Fellow working on a historical study of American medicine, suggests that the surplus of doctors said to be already upon us may offer solutions to the problem of maldistribution.

Is medical care a citizen's right? If so, to what does that right entitle its holder? These are questions that few people would have asked twenty years ago. Yet today, most Americans would probably agree with Max Fine, head of the Committee for National Health Insurance, who has written: "Americans have a right to good health care. It is not a privilege to which some should be entitled and others not. It is not a luxury to be rationed according to one's ability to pay. It is not a commodity whose priority of purchase an individual family can determine along with cars, boats, CB radios and stereo sets."

The problem, of course, is fulfilling that right. As Benjamin B. Page, an assistant professor of philosophy and health services administration, explains in the final article in this section, no society has ever provided unlimited medical services to all its citizens. If attempted, delivering those services could use up a good portion of a nation's budget, leaving little for other socially valuable programs such as education.

Nonetheless, a growing segment of the US population has begun to demand medical care as a right—and to expect the government to advance and protect that right. Through Medicaid, Medicare, and other programs, the government has taken steps in the direction of meeting the demand. The concept of medical care as a right informs the move toward national health insurance and adds a sense of urgency to any discussion of medical care in America. Indeed, the concept has become a basic issue in the movement to reshape America's medical-care system.

HEALTH CARE AND THE PATIENT'S NEEDS [1]

The major trends in medicine in the United States in recent decades have led to increasing scientific research, the specialization of physicians, and the development of an elaborate technology for the diagnosis and treatment of disease. These developments have resulted in a greatly increased understanding of disease processes and significant advances in the treatment of many serious problems. Unfortunately, they have also caused some fundamental imbalances between the kinds of medical care that are available and the needs of patients; coupled with an emphasis on free

[1] From article by Mary W. Herman, assistant professor of community health and preventive medicine, Jefferson Medical College, Philadelphia. *Current History.* 73:1–4+. Jl./Ag. '77. Copyright © 1977 by Current History, Inc. Reprinted by permission.

enterprise, they have also produced cost increases that exceed those of any other sector of the economy. In terms of the system's impact on the health of its citizens, concentration on the treatment of disease rather than the maintenance of health may well be the most serious deficiency in the present allocation of resources. . . .

In addition, all segments of the population are not equally well covered by health insurance, and major gaps remain in the kinds of services that are covered by insurance. Although almost 90 percent of the population have insurance for hospital and surgical care, only about one third are covered for physicians' services provided in the office or home. Preventive services, routine eye and dental services, drugs and appliances (including such commonly needed appliances as eyeglasses) are seldom covered by health insurance. Coverage for mental health services is usually very limited.

Medicaid now pays for the medical care of many of the most needy families, but others with low incomes lack private health insurance and are not eligible for public assistance. In 1970, for example, only 40 percent of the households with family incomes of less than $3,000 had hospital insurance. Individuals in the poorest paid occupations are also least likely to have health insurance as part of their total benefit package. In many states, Medicaid is restricted to households that are dependent on public welfare, and the adequacy of its pay schedules and the comprehensiveness of its coverage vary greatly throughout the country. As medical costs have escalated, the most common solution has been to reduce the size of the population eligible for Medicaid and to set limits on the fees that will be paid. Many elderly people are also poor or living on limited incomes. The general inflation and rapidly rising costs of Medicare premiums, copayment requirements when medical care is used, and uncovered services and drugs cause many financial hardships to this group, whose need for medical care is great.

The unequal insurance coverage of different aspects of

medical care costs leads to two major types of problems. For those with limited incomes, high costs deter individuals from seeking medical care early when treatment is likely to be more effective and less costly; and less pressing problems, such as dental and eye-care needs, may be neglected altogether. At all income levels, the more complete insurance coverage of hospital care has encouraged both doctors and patients to favor hospital utilization wherever feasible, even if the treatment would be equally effective in a doctor's office or a hospital outpatient department.

Unequal coverage also appears to have contributed to considerable unnecessary surgery. Although the figures may be a little high, a recent congressional survey concluded on the basis of sample data that as many as 2.4 million unnecessary surgical procedures were performed in 1974, which resulted in 11,900 deaths. . . .

Availability of Medical Care

Since World War II there have been many signs that there were insufficient numbers of physicians available to meet the growing demands for service. Since 1950, however, the number of medical schools in the United States has increased from 79 to 114, and many schools have increased the size of their student bodies. As a result, the overall physician-population ratio has been rising and is expected to reach adequate levels by 1980. By the 1970s, there was general agreement that the major problem was no longer the total supply of physicians but the declining number of generalists or primary care physicians and the uneven distribution of physicians geographically.

Although the trend toward specialization in medicine is not a recent development, the proportion of medical graduates entering specialty training or engaging in restricted practices has increased greatly since the 1930s. The effects have been cumulative and are continuing, because general practitioners are now concentrated in the older age groups. In 1973, general practitioners constituted only 17 percent of all physicians. Specialists in internal medicine and pediatrics are the other major sources of primary care, but most graduate training programs in these specialties are not designed to train physicians for primary care, and increasing proportions of physicians certified in these areas are engaged in specialty care.

The shift to specialization among medical graduates is a response to the increasing complexity of medical knowledge and technology, in combination with the higher incomes and prestige within the profession associated with medical specialization, teaching and research. It also reflects the kinds of students selected for admission to medical schools and the nature of their training, much of which occurs within teaching hospitals that are centers for the treatment of the more serious and esoteric conditions. The physicians being produced in turn tend to rely heavily on the sophisticated technology found in hospitals in their practice and to focus on the technical rather than the social or human side of medicine.

In 1969, a new specialty of family medicine was established to train physicians specifically for primary care and to improve the earning potential and status of generalist physicians. The number of residencies in family medicine increased rapidly; by 1974, there were 219 residencies in this specialty, which attracted 20 percent of all medical graduates in that year. Efforts are also being directed toward the development of more suitable training programs for general internists and general pediatricians. Legislative pressure is being applied through the Health Professions Educational Assistance Act of 1976, which ties medical school subsidies (capitation payments) to schools to having some minimum proportion of their residents in general internal medicine, general pediatrics, and family medicine.

The trend toward specialization has also led to a reduction in the proportion of physicians engaged in direct patient care and an increase in the proportion of those with hospital- rather than office-based practices. Between 1963 and 1973, the proportion of physicians engaged primarily in patient care declined from almost 90 to 80 percent. The number of physicians with office-based practices declined from 65 to 55 percent of all physicians. Many office-based practitioners are also found near hospitals. Those with specialty practices, in particular, settle primarily in areas with larger population concentrations, with the result that by 1973 there were 172 physicians per 100,000 population in metropolitan areas but only 79 per 100,000 in nonmetropolitan areas.

A direct relationship is also found between the economic level of an area and its supply of physicians. Doctors, like other people with relatively high incomes, are attracted to areas with good housing and schools and congenial neighbors; and unlike most employed people, they have considerable freedom in choosing where they will settle. Because of the unfavorable living and working conditions found in urban ghettos, these areas and isolated rural areas have the greatest dearth of office-based practitioners. Dwellers in the inner-city areas may not be far removed physically from excellent medical technology in nearby hospitals and medical centers, but this delivery system is in many ways the least appropriate for persons of low income and low educational attainment. Even physical access may be difficult for those living beyond walking distance.

Along with the decline in primary care practitioners, the number of patients seen per week has risen, and there has been a marked increase in the use of ambulatory services in hospitals, especially the emergency department.

Despite the declining proportion of physicians in office-based practices, this is still the source of most ambulatory care. Group practices have been growing rapidly in number, but most of them are relatively small and the physicians in them work in much the same way that solo practitioners do. Under the small group or solo practice system, medical care is a private matter between the individual physician and his patients, subject to little oversight or control by other members of the profession. Physicians in larger, multispecialty groups and those with hospital-based practices are more likely to engage in frequent exchanges of information and are subject to much more rigorous scrutiny by their peers. Since a patient is poorly equipped to evaluate the technical quality of care provided, colleague controls over physician performance are essential for assuring reasonable standards of care.

The aspect of patient care that is most likely to suffer in larger group practices is the quality of the physician-patient relationship and the physician's responsiveness to the patient's concerns and convenience. This appears to result both from the greater dominance of professional opinion that stresses the technical aspects of medicine and, in some cases, from the development of rigid bureaucratic structures. The latter are particularly characteristic of hospital clinics, which developed primarily as training sites and sources of care for indigent patients. The sustaining aspects of medical care are also likely to be neglected by overworked physicians who allow little time per patient visit. Allowing nurses, nurse practitioners and physicians' assistants to provide many aspects of patient care that traditionally are restricted to physicians would help relieve pressures on physicians. Many studies have demonstrated that less highly trained health workers can safely carry out many routine aspects of patient care, are in many cases better able than physicians to communicate with patients and meet their needs for emotional support, and are usually acceptable to patients whether they are working in small or large group practices. The organization of medical care delivery is under the direction of physicians, however, and thus far they have shown little tendency to make effective use of such practitioners. . . .

Treatment of Common Medical Problems

Perhaps the major discrepancy between the needs of patients and the kinds of medical care available is illustrated by the sort of problems for which the services of a physician are most commonly sought. These include upper respiratory infections, mild to moderate psychiatric and psychosocial problems, simple injuries, skin problems, allergies, a variety of other infections, hypertension, ulcers, asthma, malignancies, arthritis, diabetes mellitus, and obesity. Among young children a large proportion of visits to doctors are made for health check-ups and immunizations.

Many of these problems are self-limiting in nature and/ or are problems about which most doctors feel they can do very little. Others are chronic problems requiring routine management for the most part. Clearly, first-contact medical care requires good diagnostic competence that leads to an early recognition of serious problems, but it also requires a broad view of problems and interest in patients and their concerns. At present, training directed to producing physicians capable of performing these functions is largely limited to family practice residencies. Patients with common, minor ailments, especially those with psychological problems, are likely to receive inappropriate care and may even be perceived as nuisances by a busy physician. The authors of one study of a primary care practice concluded that 40 to 50 percent of the work being done could be transferred to less highly trained health personnel working in a team arrangement with physicians.

Fragmentation of Patient Care

The other major problem associated with the trend toward specialization in medicine is the fragmentation and depersonalization of patient care. With the increasing scarcity of primary care practitioners, individuals at all economic levels frequently have no personal physician or regular source of medical care to which they turn first when a problem arises. The lack of continuity between doctors (or health-care providers) and patients is detrimental both to the physician's understanding of the patient's problems and to the sense of satisfaction which both are likely to have with the relationship. Symptoms can be better understood if a patient's history and way of life are known and, given the time constraints under which most medical care is provided, this is likely only when a continuing relationship develops. Continuity also greatly increases the potential for communication and understanding between doctor and patient, factors closely related to patient satisfaction and willingness to comply with the recommended treatment. Finally, a regular source of medical care is related to seeking treatment promptly when symptoms develop.

Whether medical care is received from a number of different specialists, as is common among patients from higher income levels, or from a combination of private practitioners, outpatient clinics and emergency services, as is more common among lower income households, duplication of tests and uncoordinated care are likely to result. In addition, some bias in the type of treatment the patient is likely to receive is inherent in the specialty of the physician chosen. The relatively large supply of surgeons in the United States, for example, is generally believed to be related to the higher rate of surgery found in this country. Specialists also tend to rely heavily on elaborate and expensive diagnostic tests and procedures, which may not represent optimal care in terms of an overall concept of costs and effectiveness.

Hospital clinics are generally organized along specialty lines; responsibility for a given patient's care is divided among a number of practitioners and changes over time; and most clinics are available only at limited hours. The emergency service is designed to provide neither comprehensive nor continuing care, but is increasingly being utilized by patients from all walks of life when their regular physician or clinic is not available, and may be the only source of medical care for significant numbers of low-income households. Because of the extensive and increasing use of hospital ambulatory services, they are seen by some as an important source of much future ambulatory care; a number of hospitals are reorganizing these services so that continuing and comprehensive care can be provided in a manner responsive to patients' needs and preferences.

Although for many years health education has been regarded as a function of personal medical care as well as a component of community health services, it has received relatively minor attention and financial support. As the cost of treating disease and pressures on the available sources of medical care mount, however, public attention is increasingly being directed to the importance of education for disease prevention, the appropriate use of services, and self-care by laymen.

Behavioral contributions to such major health problems as lung cancer, coronary heart disease, alcoholism, drug addictions, and automobile accidents suggest that health education has a significant potential for reducing both the medical care costs and the human suffering that result from these conditions. Thoughtful physicians believe that the identification of risk factors and preventive health education are essential aspects of good medical care, although they are frequently neglected. There is also considerable interest in developing more effective community health education and behavioral modification programs directed to disease prevention. Because much basic information on the behavioral causes of major health problems is already widely known and because the behavior involved is imbedded in the American culture and economy, education alone may have only limited effects. Regulation and taxation of harmful products, like automobiles and cigarettes, and changes in attitudes toward individual responsibility for avoiding preventable diseases are probably necessary before any significant changes occur.

Health-care providers should also be an important source of education to patients under their care, but available evidence indicates that communication between doctors and patients is frequently very limited. Good patient care requires a discussion of the patient's concerns and the provision of information on the nature of his condition, the reasons for the proposed treatment, and its likely effects. When this is done, patients can make more informed choices and are more likely to comply with the treatment. Health-care providers can also assist patients in making more appropriate use of their services through education on the significance of symptoms, problems they can care for themselves, and when the services of experts are required. Patients with chronic conditions need medical supervision, but can participate actively in their own care when adequate information and counseling are provided.

Another important problem for the consumer is finding an appropriate source of care. Except for a few directories providing only limited information, when medical care is needed almost no assistance is available to the consumer in selecting a physician or hospital. Most physicians are reluctant to encourage consumer education and counseling for this purpose. But given the diversity in the quality and types of medical care available and the differences in consumer preferences, resources must be developed to make possible more informed choices with respect to the point of entry into the medical care system.

Other Preventive Services

The control of environmental pollution, immunizations, and programs for the early detection of disease are also important components of a comprehensive program for disease prevention. Although programs for the control of environmental pollution are administratively outside the medical care system, they play an important role in preventing a number of major health problems and they may be one of the most important factors in the control of many cancers. Immunizations and vaccinations have largely eradicated formerly common diseases like diphtheria, measles and poliomyelitis, but unfortunately these diseases are beginning to appear again in increasing numbers as more children are not protected against them in early childhood.

The value of screening populations for the early detection of disease is less generally agreed upon. The cost per case of disease discovered is frequently high, and in many cases early detection has not led to effective intervention. Screening programs directed to high-risk populations, however, and related to assured access to medical care when indicated can lead to earlier and more effective treatment for such serious health problems as cervical cancer, hypertension (and the coronary heart disease and strokes that are related to it) and glaucoma. Comprehensive periodic health examinations can also have a significant impact on the health of populations if appropriately directed to high-risk groups and related to treatment. Physicians in private practice can also play an important role in the early detection of disease among the patients and families of patients under their care.

With the increased financial support available for health services to the poor through Medicare and Medicaid, the utilization rates for physicians' services among low-income populations have risen above those of higher income levels. The poor continue to show significantly higher rates of illness and disability, however, and utilization indexes based on the need for medical care show lower use of services by the poor than other groups. Other signs of inequity are the still higher disability rates among poor nonwhites and their lower utilization of physicians' services. Although many of the causes of these less favorable indexes of health status lie outside the functions of the medical care system, barriers to the effective use of services are part of the problem.

Deficiencies in the Medicare and Medicaid programs and the inadequate availability of medical care in low-income areas have been mentioned. Studies of Medicaid programs have indicated considerable abuse of the system both by providers and users and (especially among physicians and clinics catering to this clientele) the provision of poor quality care. Cultural differences between providers and low-income clients and the bureaucratic organization of services at most hospital outpatient departments also act as barriers to the appropriate use of services and to good doctor-patient relationships. Reorganization of hospital and ambulatory services may help to alleviate the problem, but neighborhood health centers oriented to ethnic and racial neighborhood populations will apparently continue to be needed in many low-income areas, despite the problems that have been associated with them.

Services for the Elderly and Chronically Ill

More people are living longer to an age when their needs for medical care and for assistance with personal care and the activities of daily living rapidly increase. In addition, many younger people also require long-term care. These include the mentally ill and retarded and those with other chronic illnesses and physical disabilities. For individuals who cannot care for themselves, the major alternatives available today are care by members of their own families or institutional care. Relatively little assistance is available to families who undertake this care, and, increasingly, either there is no close relative or the family is unable or unwilling to care for the elderly and disabled. Nursing homes and other institutions for the long-term care of the elderly have increased rapidly since 1966, and now account for more than 60 percent of all inpatient beds in the United States.

Although there is great variability in the quality of care provided in institutions for long-term care, many are little more than custodial warehouses, providing neither necessary services nor humane attention. Most institutions for the chronically ill and retarded are publicly owned and suffer from a severe shortage of funds. As a result, their professional staffs are limited in number, and much direct patient care is undertaken by poorly paid aides, many of whom are not well suited to this type of work. Although the number of patients in psychiatric hospitals has been sharply reduced as the result of new medicines and community mental health programs, conditions in these institutions have not greatly improved. Most elderly people in institutions live in nursing homes, 80 percent of which are privately owned. The quality of care found in them, while highly variable, is also poor in all too many cases.

The care of the chronically ill and elderly could be improved by the application of stricter standards of quality control, which should be feasible since many operate under public auspices or depend heavily on public funds, Medicare, Medicaid and Social Security. Another more important policy decision would be to encourage the development of more adequate programs designed to permit individuals needing care to continue to live in private homes, alone, with their own families, or with others in the community. Home health services, personal services and financial support to households providing this care would be required, but would probably be a less expensive and more humane way to meet the needs of those requiring long-term care.

In the wake of rapid expansion in medical knowledge and technology, the American health-care system has developed major imbalances between specialty and primary care, in its distribution of facilities and physicians, and in its emphasis on the technical side of disease treatment rather than on the sustaining aspects of medical care or the prevention of disease. Health insurance and public support for the care of the most needy segments of the population have reduced some inequities but have ignored other inequities and have contributed to the inflationary spiral of medical care costs. Although programs have been developed that demonstrate some of the ways in which medical care delivery could be made more efficient and effective, no overall policies that would overcome the nation's major health-care problems have yet been determined. It is clear, however, that only a broad view of the causes, control, and treatment of disease and disability will lead to a substantial impact without an unreasonable allocation of resources to the health sector of the economy.

WHY RURAL DOCTORS ARE MISSING [2]

For years we have heard about the nationwide crisis in the health-care system, but while some improvement has taken place in urban and suburban areas, the situation has only worsened in the countryside.

[2] Article entitled "The Rural Health Care Crisis," by John B. Dunne, executive director, Connecticut Valley Health Compact, a New Hampshire–Vermont health planning agency. *Blair & Ketchum's Country Journal.* 3:71–7. Ap. '76. Reprinted by permission from *Blair & Ketchum's Country Journal.* Copyright © 1976, Country Journal Publishing Company.

Many examples could be presented, but let's look at one rural county in Pennsylvania. In the northern part of this county is a town with a sixty-bed hospital. Six physicians staff this facility and provide medical care for the several thousand people. Four of these physicians are over sixty-five, and one of the younger ones has had his first coronary. A mobile health-screening unit was sent into the area for six months. Five thousand persons who were screened on the unit had not seen a doctor in five years. There were diabetic, hypertensive, cardiac, renal, and other seriously ill patients. They might as well have been living in the Andes Mountains as far as contact with medical care is concerned. If this is true in a populous industrial state, how much more critical is it in Vermont, Maine, Idaho, Arkansas, or Kentucky?

One of the most pressing problems is attracting physicians to rural areas and keeping them there. Several factors are involved here:

A. *Excessive patient load, so the doctor may have to work all the time.* A common complaint of many rural physicians is that they don't have any time they can call their own. One doctor living in a town of 4,000 people said he had a patient load of 5,500—people who came from outside of town by the dozens. He said he had to refuse to take any more patients, because when he took a man or his wife as a patient, he usually inherited the family and thus, in fact, added four or five altogether. Like many other physicians in similar circumstances, he works an average of 75 to 80 hours a week. He said he would gladly pay another physician handsomely to share the load but had been unable to find any takers.

B. *Lack of sophisticated equipment and technical assistance.* This often affects young physicians who choose to open an office in a rural area. Most doctors receive their education in medical centers where they have ultramodern equipment to aid in diagnosis, treatment, and rehabilitation of patients. In the country they are faced with large numbers of patients with diverse complaints and symptoms and relatively little in the way of sophisticated equipment to assist them. In the medical center they could also request laboratory tests, X-rays, radio-isotope scans, electroencephalograms, and so on, and a skilled physician or technician would perform the service and advise the physician of the findings. Such assistance is not available in the country. The doctor learns very early in his practice that he has to improvise and make do.

C. *Spouse and family dissatisfaction.* A few years ago many physicians married a home-town girl after returning from medical school. She knew the people, was used to the tempo of the town or village, participated in local activities, and was generally satisfied to occupy a position of some prominence as the doctor's wife in a small community. Contrast that with what happens so often today. The medical student or intern or resident meets and marries a young woman from the city in which the medical school is located. If he moves to a rural area, he brings his bride to a new way of life in which the week's excitement may be a band concert at the high school, a basketball game, or a bake sale. The movie house is open on Friday and Saturday and may be featuring *Gone With the Wind* or a revival of *Andy Hardy*. If the doctor's wife is interested in working, there aren't many opportunities. Meanwhile, her husband is kept so busy with his growing patient load that he has a minimum of time for his wife or family.

D. *Lack of opportunities for continuing education.* The complaint has been made that some physicians haven't opened a book since they finished medical school. Generally speaking, this is untrue. Many doctors have a thirst for more knowledge about their profession. They may read copiously from a number of journals, but this does not take the place of some formalized continuing education. While ample opportunities are available in the cities, often there are few or none in the small towns. This is especially true in winter, when driving may be treacherous enough to make attending sessions impractical. This dearth of mental stimulation is anathema to a conscientious physician, but many have to accept it as a fact of rural practice. In answering a recent questionnaire concerning what they felt was most needed to improve patient care, an overwhelming number of physicians with rural practices answered "continuing education courses."

E. *Distance from hospitals makes referrals difficult and precludes learning experiences.* The rural physician learns to keep his patients as well as he can with adequate medication and personal follow-up. There are cases, however, that need hospitalization. If the doctor has staff privileges at the nearest hospital, he may elect to send the patient there. If he knows that the patient requires treatment that the small hospital cannot provide, he will send the patient to the nearest medical center, which may be fifty or so miles away. Either alternative is less than ideal. The patient cannot be seen by his physician on a regular basis in the community hospital if it is some distance away, and unless the rural doctor knows specialists in the medical center to whom he can refer his patient, the patient may get lost in the shuffle. The doctor might not see the patient again until the patient is in a critical state. (This is especially true in cancer cases.) Too few rural physicians have an opportunity to practice in a hospital and they miss it sorely.

F. *Students from rural areas seldom return to their home towns to practice.* One would asume that a logical source of physicians would be resident young people who go to medical school. Unfortunately, this is not the case. The lure of the large center where he or she receives medical education—or perhaps the hospital where a residency is served—often serves as a magnet. Even if the student had every intention of returning to his community, the intervening years bring changes, and the hopes of the home town are dashed.

G. *Unfriendly attitude of established physicians.* It might seem that established physicians in a rural area would welcome the arrival of help on the scene in the person of a young physician, but often this is not the case. The new arrival may find a chilly reception from his peers. The older ones may be willing and eager to pass along to the new doctor their chronic complainers, hypochondriacs, and stroke patients. Sometimes, of course, this boomerangs because a young, knowledgeable physician may really help some of these patients and establish a reputation as a fine doctor.

H. *Adequate remuneration often fails to compensate for disadvantages.* A common fallacy is that the easiest way to assure an adequate supply of physicians in rural areas is to hold out the promise of a lucrative practice. Some communities have gone to some pains to guarantee an incoming physician a good income and have even provided an attractive clinic in which he can practice. Under these seemingly ideal circumstances, the doctor may arrive and engage in practice for a year or two and then depart. The stunned citizens of the community are at a loss to know what happened. Perhaps a review of the problems outlined above would shed some light on their dilemma.

Community Options Open

The problem, as I have tried to suggest, is grave. Thousands of rural citizens have inadequate medical care or none at all. Scores of communities have seen their only doctor succumb to a heart attack or move away, and these towns and villages have no replacement physician.

While there is no single easy solution, there are at least a number of options available to the community in search of a doctor. Here are some of them:

A. *National Health Service Corps.* The Department of Health, Education, and Welfare has developed a plan to provide physicians to underserved areas in urban and rural settings. This program—the National Health Service Corps —works with physicians who do not wish to carry out their service obligation. Obviously, the matter of fitting the right physician to the right community is extremely important. If the area to be served feels that the doctor, because of urban training and orientation, is not sympathetic to their problems, the situation can be very sticky. If, on the other hand, the professional feels that he has been assigned to "nowheresville," the period of his service will not be a happy one. The community may at last have a doctor to serve its needs, but his service may be grudging and unsatisfactory.

On the other hand, if the placement is a good one, both physician and community can profit for the two years he is there. There is always the chance that he will like it so well, and be liked so well, that he will settle in as the area physician when his period in the Health Service Corps is up. As a footnote, it should be said that if the National Health Service Corps is to be successful in helping solve the rural health-care delivery problem, it must have adequate, not minimal, funding and be staffed by persons with dedication and imagination—those who have personally investigated the needs of the rural population in the health-care field.

B. *Physician's Assistants.* The acceptance of paramedical persons to perform many of the services formerly performed by doctors has not been universially enthusiastic in rural areas. In some communities, the physician's assistant has been looked upon as a poor substitute for the longed-for family doctor. In other areas, however, these well-trained people have been welcomed and have established a level of excellent primary care. There are at present a number of variations of physician's assistants. There are returned veterans with a background in the armed services' medical corps; they are known as medics, and generally work under a physician preceptor after a period of training. There are nurse practitioners who are RNs with special training in a medical center to prepare them to serve as assistants under a preceptor physician. There are nurse-midwives who are specially trained by obstetricians to take responsibility for prenatal care, delivery, and postnatal care in normal childbirth cases. There are medex assistants who can be recruited from any of the paramedical specialties and given intensive training before being entrusted with routine patient health problems.

The receptiveness to physician's assistants by physicians and medical societies has varied. In the state of Washington and elsewhere in the Northwest, the physician's assistants generally function well under physician preceptors. In Kentucky, the nurse-midwife has for many years been an integral part of the health-care system in rural areas.

As these people are used more widely, we will be able to assess their impact on rural health care, but even as of now it is clear that a well-trained, highly motivated physician's assistant can do many of the things that until recently only MDs were thought capable of doing.

C. *The Physician's Spouse and Children.* As noted above, a dissatisfied family plays a significant role in the doctor's decision to leave a community. Frequently, it takes only a little extra effort on the part of a community to see that his family is accepted and integrated into the local scene. All too often a great effort is made to recruit a physician, only to let his wife and children shift for themselves in an unfamiliar atmosphere. No community can be assured that its physician is going to remain if his family is neglected.

D. *Continuing Education Program for Physicians.* Recent years have seen innovations in postgraduate medical education, including dial-a-program, closed-circuit television, audio-visual tape programs, and audio tapes—many of them designed to reach the rural physician. Unfortunately, most such systems rely on the doctor's watching or listening or both, but do not require his participation, do not permit him to question or express an opinion. And without such interaction, the effectiveness of such programs is jeopardized. Now, the University of Vermont Medical School and Dartmouth Medical School jointly offer a TV program that permits participation by doctors.

A dynamic continuing education program includes lectures, panels, case presentation, patient rounds, and peer review—all activities involving the physician. There are also regional medical programs that bring faculty members into small communities in rural areas, expanding the universities' role as dynamic forces in the life of an area. However it comes about, there is probably no better way to provide job satisfaction for the rural physician than to make it easier for him to continue learning medicine.

E. *Preceptor Programs for the Rural Physician.* The University of West Virginia Medical School inaugurated an innovative program some years ago. It involves having a physician from the university cover the practice of a rural physician, while the latter goes to the university to work with patients in the medical center. A preceptor is available to see that the rural doctor gets the needed exposure to meaningful cases. Reports indicate a high level of enthusiasm for this program on the part of both the rural physician and the university doctor. It is another important educational back-up for the rural physician.

F. *Internships and Residencies in Family Medicine.* For many years, the medical community has regarded an internship as a glorified apprenticeship served by the new physician in a teaching hospital. Certain internships were considered more prestigious than others, because a greater mix of patients could be seen. For a few years, interns in Kansas have been encouraged to work with family practitioners in small communities and rural areas. This system provides added medical manpower and allows the young doctor to develop skill and resourcefulness. Hahnemann Medical School in Philadelphia has a similar program, and other medical schools are planning rural intern or resident programs. This experience offers the doctor an opportunity to observe primary medical care and also to practice the skills he has learned in school. And there is always the chance that the young physician will develop ties with the community that will influence his choice of a place to practice.

A fairly recent development of significance to the manpower problem in the rural area is a program instituted by the University of Minnesota School of Medicine. Third-year medical students are sent into small towns under the Rural Physicians Associate Program. Under the program the students receive a salary of $10,000 for the year—half of it paid by a grant from the legislature and half by the local physician for whom the student works. The physicians who have agreed to participate are enthusiastic about the program; it not only gives the prospective physician confidence but also increases his knowledge about the actual practice of family medicine.

G. *Involvement in Health Planning.* A law passed in January 1975, called the National Health Planning and Resources Development Act, requires the states to designate certain health service areas and a health systems agency as a means to formulating a comprehensive health plan. The success of the act obviously depends on input from rural as well as urban areas. The rural doctor can take a leadership role in these agencies and indeed, by working with committed consumers and other professionals, can help to bring about improved health care. By participating in such a program, the rural doctor can enunciate the needs of his area and may request grant money to implement continuing education programs and provide outreach clinics.

H. *Scholarship Programs.* Some country medical societies offer scholarships to college graduates from the area who wish to enter medical school and who are accepted. Some of the scholarships require that the recipient return to that county to practice for a specified period after becoming a physician. Such a program does not alleviate the present acute shortage, but it will eventually provide a manpower pool of young doctors. Some communities have also discovered that it pays to interest their young people in the health services as early as possible by having local professionals counsel high school students on what is involved in becoming a doctor or a nurse, or in going into physical therapy or another branch of medicine.

I. *Recruitment Programs.* A hospital in a rural town in western Pennsylvania has developed a sophisticated recruitment program to attract physicians to the area. It goes something like this. A physician and his spouse are invited to fly into the county airport at the expense of the recruitment committee. They are put up at the best motel. A dinner is held for them at the country club, and they are introduced to resident physicians and their spouses. The next day the prospective doctor is given a tour of the hospital and asked to make rounds. In the meantime a committee of the medical society auxiliary takes his spouse on a tour of churches and schools, discusses available employment and other matters of interest. While this is going on, the doctor is conferring with other physicians who are evaluating him as he sizes them up. If the search or recruitment committee is properly impressed, they invite the doctor to come to the area to practice. They offer him a guaranteed income for a year and, if necessary, a program to assist him to purchase a home.

Other Programs Available

In addition to the specific problems and specific solutions cited here, consideration should be given to programs now in effect or proposed that may help to alleviate the health-care crisis in rural areas.

HMO Concept. The initials HMO stand for Health Maintenance Organization, which is a program of prepaid comprehensive group health care. The objective of such an organization goes beyond caring for patients during and after an illness; an attempt is made to keep members well through screening, health examinations, and early detection of symptoms. Hospitalization, emergency care, and outpatient services are also provided in return for a predetermined monthly fee for members. An HMO can serve a rural area through outreach clinics or health centers, staffed by physician's assistants, nurse practitioners, and other paramedical personnel. Physicians from the central health center of the HMO make scheduled visits to these rural centers and see patients who need a physician's attention. The member thus served also has access to services in the health center. Usually, prescriptions are provided at cost, or free. In the event of an emergency, the patient can call the health center at any hour of any day of the week and be directed what to do.

Home health care is provided by visiting nurses so that the patient's recovery in the home is enhanced. . . . [For additional information about HMOs see Section VI, below.]

Community Health Councils. It is not always possible to embrace the HMO concept in sparsely settled areas. Here, instead, councils can be established by citizens with the aim of establishing a full-service health clinic. In Londonderry, Vermont, such a council was recently organized with the help of the Dartmouth Medical School Department of Community Medicine and the Connecticut Valley Health Compact, an areawide health planning agency. Citizens of towns around Londonderry got together and formed a nonprofit corporation; a fund-raising drive produced more than $150,000; and ground was broken for a health center in May 1975. This center will have facilities for one to three doctors, a nurse practitioner, paramedical personnel, and visiting nurse and mental health personnel.

Mobile Health Units. The success of a mobile unit depends on how well it is staffed, what services it can perform, and the frequency of its appearance in small, doctorless communities. If a mobile health unit provides only screening and examination services it may do more harm than good. Certainly it will find many untreated patients and uncover unsuspected pathology, but if these patients cannot be included in the health-care delivery system, expectations have been raised only to be let down again. To render a real service, the mobile unit must make regular visits and provide needed medications, therapy, and even rehabilitation.

Home Health-Care Program. Visiting nurse programs have provided excellent care to homebound patients in urban areas for many years. The stroke patient, the patient recently discharged from the hospital, the diabetic or cardiac patient have all benefited from the care administered by these nurses. In recent years, the service of the visiting nurse has been augmented by the home health-care aide. Thanks to the cooperation between some regional medical programs and existing visiting nurse associations, services have been expanded to include rural counties. One such program now operates in Cambria, Bedford, and Somerset counties in central Pennsylvania. The leadership and supervision for this was provided by the Johnstown Visiting Nurse Association; home health-aides were trained, the supervisory staff was expanded, and the service was made available to previously under-served villages and boroughs. The residents of one small town painted and refurnished an abandoned two-room school house for the nurse's office. Modest charges to patients and insurance payments for services have made this almost self-supporting.

The health-care crisis that exists in rural America is a problem that defies easy solutions—but it is not insoluble. It will, however, require the best efforts of local communities, counties, states, the medical schools, and the federal government. If health care is the right of every American, we must find the will and the means to make the health-care system work in rural America. Complacency will have to give way to imaginative, innovative, bold, and even untried programs, if we are to solve the problem that plagues every rural county in our land.

TOO MANY DOCTORS? [3]

Some changes pass over institutions slowly. For a while they go unrecognized, only gradually coming into plain view, until suddenly we realize that things are not nearly the same as we remember them. So it will be, I think, with a little noticed but highly significant development in medicine—the great expansion of medical education since 1965 and the now rapidly increasing supply of physicians.

Strange as it may seem to people who still can't find a

[3] Article, "A Coming Doctor Surplus?" by Paul Starr, editor. *Working Papers for a New Society.* 4:18–19+. Winter '77. Reprinted by permission of Working Papers for a New Society; © 1977 Center for the Study of Public Policy, Inc.

doctor on weekends, much less get a house call anytime, there is serious talk now about an impending "doctor surplus" after years of lament over a "doctor shortage." Measures have even been proposed to hold down the number of new physicians. With remarkably little fanfare, Congress has already taken one step in that direction. Yet the momentum of expansion in medical education seems irresistible well into the 1980s, and the political and economic implications of a flood of new doctors could be profound. For reasons I'll come to shortly, I see this as one of the most promising developments in medicine today, but conceivably it could aggravate our problems, or perhaps come to nothing.

The facts are striking. Within the past decade, the yearly increase in the number of new physicians has doubled. The sources have been both foreign and domestic. Foreign medical graduates admitted to the country as immigrants rose from just 2,000 a year in 1965 to more than 7,000 by 1972. Graduates of US medical schools climbed from 7,500 in 1966 to 13,000 last spring [1976] as a result of increases in both the size and number of schools. Ten years ago there were 88 medical schools; now there are 114, with 13 more being planned. If these are completed as scheduled, the total increase since 1966 will amount to almost 40 new medical schools—this in a country that had hardly seen any net growth at all during the previous half century.

Because population growth has slowed, the gains in the supply of doctors relative to population are quite impressive. The number of physicians per 100,000 people in America grew from 148 in 1960 to 174 in 1975; by 1985, according to recent projections, it will soar to between 210 and 218. At that point, probably only Israel and the Soviet Union will have proportionately more physicians than the United States. Today, in training, there are almost a third as many doctors in America (roughly 100,000) as there are in active practice. When current medical students and residents inundate the market, the effects should be enormous.

The likely availability of large numbers of new doctors

could greatly facilitate future efforts to change the medical system. Young physicians, just coming out of medical school without any prior attachment to private, fee-for-service practice, may be more readily attracted to new institutions and arrangements than older physicians. There is some evidence that the new graduates, particularly women, are less interested than their predecessors in setting themselves up as solo entrepreneurs. But whatever their preferences, they may find it increasingly difficult to get started in private practice, which now, especially because of rising malpractice insurance rates and medical equipment costs, requires an investment beyond the reach of many young doctors. Instead, they may turn to neighborhood clinics, health maintenance organizations [see Section VI, below] and other institutions that offer secure salaries. The fee-for-service system will most likely be changed, not by making old docs do new tricks, but by generating large numbers of new physicians who find it in their interest to accept arrangements that established practitioners would shun.

A large and expanding supply of physicians also offers a new opportunity to alter the balance of power in medicine. The strength of the medical profession in America has long rested on its success in restricting its own numbers. By holding down the supply of physicians, the organized profession has been able to maintain the highest median income of any occupation, and to defeat programs and institutions that threaten its interests. Because of opposition from medical societies, consumer-sponsored health plans, in various forms, have typically found it almost impossible to hire staff physicians. The relative scarcity of doctors has strengthened their bargaining position with the society, enabling them to control the terms of their relationships with patients and medical institutions. Increasing the number of physicians could help reduce the profession's market power. It might even help achieve some equalization of incomes between doctors and other health workers. As Victor Fuchs [author and educator] has shown, incomes within the medical care sector have been more unequal than in any other major industry in America.

An Historical Reversal

Inroads into physicians' economic power would represent an historical reversal. Restrictions on the supply of doctors go back to the early years of the twentieth century. Through the 1880s, physicians were plentiful and, as a group, not particularly well off. Because of lax state laws, medical colleges proliferated until by 1900 there were 160 in the nation—most of them small, quick-degree, profit-making trade schools with few requirements for admission or graduation.

Successful lobbying by medical societies, however, brought stronger medical licensing laws, requiring longer periods of training, higher premedical qualifications, laboratory work, and clinical hospital instruction. Since meeting such standards cost more money than schools could raise from student tuition, medical education became unprofitable. Commercial schools closed, and almost all training was incorporated into universities. A 1910 report from the Carnegie Foundation, written by the educator Abraham Flexner, helped organize public opinion in favor of an upgraded but smaller system producing "fewer but better" doctors. By 1922 the number of medical schools had dropped from 160 to 81, and the number of graduates, which had been 5,606 in 1905, plummeted to 2,529.

While the medical schools later increased the size of their graduating classes, they grew more slowly than the nation's population. From the turn of the century through the Depression, the ratio of physicians to population dropped from 173 per 100,000 to around 130. It remained near that low level through the 1950s. In the meantime, medical services expanded enormously and specialization deepened. Between 1931 and 1963, general practitioners dwindled in number from 112,000 to 73,000, or from 72 to 28 percent of all doctors. Talk of a "doctor shortage" became common, although the country might actually have had more than enough physicians had they been rationally distributed.

The turning point came in the mid-1960s. In 1965, Congress revised the immigration laws, eliminating the old system of national quotas, which had favored European countries. Under the new law, occupations in which domestic shortages were believed to exist gained special preference. Medicine was one of these. In 1970, Congress made it easier for foreign medical students who had come here on temporary exchange visas to become permanent immigrants. As a result, the annual influx of immigrant physicians tripled by the early seventies. (Actually, many of these immigrants were already in the United States on exchange visas, but had the law not been changed, they would have found it difficult to stay.) At the same time, the major source of foreign doctors swung from Europe to Asia. Only 300 Asian doctors annually emigrated to the United States before 1965; there were 5,000 a year by 1972. India, the Philippines, and South Korea became the three major contributors in a massive redistribution of human capital from some of the poorest nations to one of the richest.

Also in the mid-sixties, the federal government undertook its first direct support for medical education. The American Medical Association (AMA), anxious to keep down the number of doctors, had long opposed such assistance, but the medical schools wanted it dearly and their influence in Washington was growing. An initial measure in 1963 provided for construction grants and student loans; in 1965, the law was amended to include funds for the schools' operating costs, on the condition that they increase enrollment a minimum amount. By the late sixties, even the AMA joined in support of federal aid for medical education after the great surge in demand for medical services resulting from the enactment of Medicare and Medicaid. Further legislation in 1968 and 1971 increased financial assistance to medical schools and strengthened the provisions making aid conditional on higher enrollments. These incentives, according to a study by RAND [Rand Corporation, a research group] were crucial in nearly doubling the number of graduates over the course of a decade.

Unbalanced Distribution

The effects of these changes have as yet scarcely been felt. It takes about eight years for increased first-year enrollments to affect the supply of doctors. Only now are the large medical school classes of the late sixties beginning to turn up on the market, and the new doctors have not yet had time to accumulate in great numbers. Among many people the impression persists that the AMA still keeps down the number of physicians, in part because one hears how difficult it is to get into medical school. (The number of applicants has increased more rapidly than the number of medical school places.) Moreover, unbalanced distribution of physicians, by region and by specialty, continues to leave shortages in rural and inner-city areas, especially in "primary care" (general and family practice, general pediatrics and internal medicine, obstetrics and gynecology). American medicine is today vastly overspecialized. In Britain, 75 percent of doctors provide primary care; in the Kaiser-Permanente health plan in America, the proportion is two thirds. [See "Kaiser and the 'Desert Doctors': A Way to Cut Medical Bills," by Lee Smith, in Section VI, below.] But in the United States as a whole, primary care accounts for only 45 percent of physicians. So, although we may be building up to a future doctor glut, genuine scarcities still exist.

A general increase in physicians provides no guarantee that these distributional problems will be resolved. Even in surplus, doctors are likely to continue to gravitate to the more prestigious and comfortable suburbs and specialties, unless there are strong incentives in other directions. Past increases have gone disproportionately to regions that already have high densities of physicians. When the supply of doctors was beginning to grow between 1963 and 1970, the proportion in primary care was actually falling. The educational system turns out highly trained specialists oriented toward work in urban settings, and the current insurance system reimburses specialists more generously for their services.

Lately, in an effort to ward off federal regulation, the AMA has been arguing that the private sector is already remedying the deficiencies in primary care. Between 1968 and 1974, the number of first-year positions in primary-care training programs jumped from 4,600 to 8,800. But the increase may be deceptive because of a growing trend toward specialization within primary-care fields. Young internists, for example, are going into subspecialties like cardiology or hematology, rather than general internal medicine. "It is almost certain," the Coordinating Council on Medical Education, a semiofficial body, stated in 1975, "that with the new opportunities for certification in subspecialties, proportionately fewer internists and pediatricians will have an interest in primary care."

New legislation passed by Congress last October [1976] makes some effort to correct these distributional problems. It requires medical schools to offer about half their residencies in primary-care fields and makes scholarships available to medical students on the condition that they work one year in doctor-poor areas for each year they receive financial aid. But in a statement of findings and policy, the law also declares that "there is no longer an insufficient number of physicians and surgeons in the United States" and, as a result, "no further need for affording preference to alien physicians and surgeons" in immigration. Further, it terminates the earlier incentives for medical schools to expand first-year classes.

Whether the law will help or hurt doctor-poor communities remains to be seen. Today, one of every five doctors in the country is a foreign medical graduate. These doctors take many of the jobs that Americans spurn, such as staffing municipal hospitals and state mental institutions. In Brooklyn, New York, more than 90 percent of the city-hospital doctors are foreign graduates. Without them, those hospitals may be in dire trouble. Until 1980, the new federal law allows exceptions to its cutoff of immigrant doctors for institutions that would be seriously disrupted by their loss. The hope is that as American medical school graduates grow in numbers, they will take the place of foreign physicians, even at the least desirable institutions.

The new scholarships are designed in part to remedy the problems caused by the loss of imported doctors. If fully funded, they will greatly augment the size of the National Health Service Corps, a federal program begun in 1972 that assigns physicians and other medical personnel to under-served areas. Until now, the corps has depended on volunteers and has placed only about two hundred doctors a year, almost entirely in rural communities. The new legislation redefines shortage areas to include public institutions, like prisons and mental hospitals, that have trouble recruiting doctors, and the corps is now preparing to move into urban neighborhoods as well as rural towns. By the mid-1980s, with the scholarships bearing fruit, the size of the program may grow to 5,000 or 10,000 doctors (some in Washington mention 20,000 as a goal). If these changes in size and orientation materialize, the National Health Service Corps could become a powerful instrument in reversing the maldistribution of doctors. Some, however, remain skeptical of a program that may end up only rotating young physicians through communities where they have no serious intention of putting down roots and establishing a practice.

Besides the cutoff of foreign medical graduates and the elimination of incentives for medical schools to expand first-year classes, other moves to slow down the expanding supply of physicians may also be in store. In a recent report, the Carnegie Council on Policy Studies—sixty-six years after Abraham Flexner—argued that the United States is now in "danger" of creating too many medical schools and called upon the federal government to abandon nearly all of the thirteen new schools now in development. Throughout the government, a consensus is apparently emerging that America is threatened with a surplus of physicians.

Policy Makers Concerned

What causes concern among policy makers is the possibility that the addition of new physicians may generate increased expenditures for medical care by driving up both the volume and the price of services. Once patients bring their complaints to a doctor, the doctor determines whether tests, operations, drugs, and further visits are necessary. These judgments are highly variable. Physicians can increase "demand" for medical services by reducing the threshold at which procedures are thought medically warranted. The higher the density of physicians in an area, the greater the pressure seems to be to perform services that otherwise might be forgone. Considerable evidence suggests that the more surgeons there are in a community, the higher the rates of surgery and hospitalization. Moreover, an increased supply of surgeons does not necessarily bring down prices. The less individual surgeons work, the more they charge, so they can keep their incomes at the levels to which they are accustomed. The economics of fee-for-service medicine seem to be completely perverse. Demand appears to be controlled by the suppliers, who raise prices to meet expected levels of income. Consequently, the rising number of doctors could quite easily inflate total medical costs for the society.

But the effects might also go the other way. A goodly supply of physicians might help prevent inflation from a national health program. Medicare and Medicaid, one often hears, pushed up medical costs because they increased demand, while the supply of physicians and facilities was relatively inelastic. Conceivably, that kind of demand-push inflation could be blunted in the future by an abundant supply of doctors.

Which of these effects will predominate is unclear. Possibly they will turn out to affect different parts of the medical system in different ways. By making doctors available at reasonable salaries, a rising supply might hold down costs for neighborhood clinics and health maintenance organizations. In the fee-for-service sector, however, more doctors will probably mean higher utilization and higher costs, forcing up the price of health insurance. The future effects of the growing supply of doctors on health-care expenditures depend fundamentally on the outlook of fee-for-service medicine. If, as I think, its prospects are poor, then the case for maintaining a high supply of doctors is correspondingly strong.

One further possibility exists. The growing supply of doctors could change the division of labor in medicine. Should physicians become more numerous and less expensive, they may displace nurse practitioners and other "physician extenders," putting an end to recent efforts to develop new paramedical occupations. They might also take over more administrative functions in the medical system. Lateral movements of this sort could prevent any surplus of doctors from developing. Don't expect to find any MDs driving taxis.

If the medical system were rationally organized in some rough relation to need, we could probably do with fewer doctors than we already have. The argument for increasing the supply is primarily political. We need more doctors who are not committed to private practice and an abundant supply of physicians to limit the economic power of the profession. At some point in the future, we may be forced into a confrontation with the medical profession over the maintenance of its privileges. Doctors' strikes over national health programs are not unheard of. At that point, it will be extremely useful to have more doctors than we need, instead of needing more doctors than we have. An expanding supply of physicians will not solve our problems, but it may create favorable objective conditions for the success of future efforts.

THE RIGHT TO HEALTH CARE [4]

There is considerable debate in the United States today over the proposition that health care is or should be considered a right. Almost every word in this proposition calls for exploration.

To begin with, there is the question of the nature and source of rights. The concept that something is or should be regarded as a right is a tool often used by those seeking to justify social change or those trying to preserve existing prerogatives in the face of efforts for change.

Both groups are active in the case of health care. On one side are the growing number of interests and groups concerned about the increasing costs of health care and the inequalities and injustices that exist in its delivery. On the other are segments of the health-care professions concerned that making health care a right would require them to practice in specialties, localities, or situations not of their own choosing. The right to health care for all, they believe, would infringe on the health-care providers' rights to free choice of how they earn their livelihoods.

Thus, in a widely read article in the *New England Journal of Medicine,* Dr. Robert W. Sade attempts to refute the proposition that health care is a right. Other health-care professionals acknowledge that there are injustices and inequalities in our society, many with a negative effect on health. But, they ask, why should the medical profession bear the brunt of efforts to correct or compensate for society's ills? Physicians are no more responsible than other elements of our society. Unless the rest of society is also to be mobilized, it is unfair, say such voices, to single out physicians as the profession whose individual rights are to be sacrificed.

Those who regard health care as a fundamental right and favor immediate action to make it available to all are

[4] Article by Benjamin B. Page, assistant professor of philosophy and health services administration, Quinniapiac College, Hamden, Connecticut. *Current History.* 73:5–8+. Jl./Ag. '77. Copyright © by Current History, Inc. Reprinted by permission.

presumably willing to accept infringement on provider rights as part of the "price" to be paid in the process. They must face a further question about the rights of care providers who would be asked to pay this price. Would physicians have the right to organize to defend their interests, perhaps even to strike, like other groups of public servants? Or is health care so basic that such provider rights would be circumscribed?

Those who stress the priority of provider rights are more likely to urge moving slowly, perhaps through the use of incentives and the like to entice providers "freely" to select needed specialties or localities. This is more in keeping with our national traditions and institutions, but it also involves a price: it means asking those now deprived in terms of access to health care to wait a while longer, in the hope that the incentives will "work."

Discussion must also focus on what it is that would be established as a right—what is health care? There is a general tendency to identify health care with medical care. Our fee-for-service system of private enterprise medicine has provided *medical* treatment to those able to pay or who are covered by appropriate insurance. To this extent "health care" has never not been a right, and those so far left out are increasingly being covered by welfare programs, Medicare, Medicaid, and the like. If this is what is meant by health care, perhaps all that is needed is the improvement of welfare coverage and mechanisms. With a guarantee of a fee for treating even the poorest patients, physicians and medical facilities might establish themselves in previously underserved poverty areas. Thus medical care would gradually become available to almost everyone, on a basis profitable to the providers of care and to their back-up in the drug and medical equipment companies. Those who could pay for it, or whose insurance could pay, would continue to be responsible themselves for health care; those who could not would become the responsibility of society through the tax and welfare systems. And all this could be accomplished with minimal government interference in the medical care system itself.

This approach raises little conflict with our established economic institutions. However, while it might entice providers to practice in heretofore underserved urban areas—as it already has, sometimes to the accompaniment of cries of "scandal" when a physician seems to be getting too rich from such practice—it would by itself do little for sparsely populated rural areas. Nor would it persuade physicians to select socially needed specialties instead of professionally interesting, prestigious or lucrative ones. Most important, it would do nothing about the problem of the cost of medical care.

Rising Medical Costs

This issue has led to a continuing debate over the financing and organization of the delivery of medical care. This debate actually began during World War I, when medical examinations for military service revealed a disturbingly large percentage of United States youth to be unfit for medical reasons, most of which could have been prevented had adequate access to adequate care been available. The Soviet revolution, the "Roaring Twenties," the Great Depression, and World War II all intervened to overshadow the problem, even though medical examinations for military service in the 1940s showed results similar to the results two and a half decades earlier.

During World War II, large numbers of servicemen and their immediate families received their first exposure to more or less regular medical care, care that was delivered under economic conditions akin to those of socialized medicine. Because of this experience, there was a strong movement after the war to nationalize medical care delivery. This movement was effectively blocked by the American Medical Association and allied interests. The upshot was the enactment of programs providing federal support for hospital construction and modernization; massive federal support for medical research (which has been responsible for the superiority of the United States in terms of technological sophistication); and the rapid expansion of private and group-based medical insurance. Because of the threat of civil violence characteristic of the early 1960s, the Administration of President Lyndon Johnson enacted several programs to improve the economic and geographical availability of medical care to minority groups and the aged.

None of these programs, however, helped to check the rising trend of medical costs, a trend caused by two factors, deeply embedded in our health-care system. One of these is the fee-for-service system. It does not matter what the source of the fees is—private patients, insurance companies, or federal programs. Most providers derive most of their income from the delivery of medical care to people suffering from illness or injury. So long as this is true, neither the providers, the hospitals and the nursing homes, nor their backup in the pharmaceutical and medical equipment industries have any *objective economic* interest in the prevention of disease or accident or in the promotion of healthful living and working conditions. In fact, the branch of medicine that deals with these issues, public health, has traditionally enjoyed far less prestige and income than have those who treat the victims of disease or accident, in the eyes of the general public and within the profession.

It is worth noting, in this regard, that the pharmaceutical and medical equipment industries have long been among the most profitable in our economy. A special issue of *Fortune* devoted to the "health-care crisis" mentioned them as major potential growth industries and hence as very good investments.

Expensive Technology

The other even more basic factor in the rising costs of medical care is the assumption that health care is equivalent to medical care, that technologically sophisticated, scientifically oriented medical care is the basis of modern health care. As in most areas, technological innovation and scientific discovery are highly costly in and of themselves.

In addition, in medicine, their application increases instead of reducing other costs. Each new procedure for diagnosis, treatment, or rehabilitation requires new capital outlays and sometimes new construction, and new categories of personnel, while it only occasionally eliminates the need for older procedures. Facilities and teachers to train new personnel must be provided; the newly trained specialists then command higher pay. Subsequent competition among providers, hospitals and nursing homes for "modernity" means that they purchase the latest equipment even if their old equipment is adequate or when there is little effective need for the new equipment.

The more technologically sophisticated but highly expensive means of diagnosis, treatment, and rehabilitation for more and more problems defined as medical problems are developed, the more the costs of medical care will rise. Costs will continue to rise if we assume that medical care is the way to realize health care as a right for all citizens, whether individual patients, insurance programs, or the state pay the bills. The Marxist countries and other countries with socialized medicine also face the problem of cost escalation.

Some Problems

Thus those who urge health care as a right and assume that making modern, scientific medical care available to all is the way to implement this right face crucial choices. As biologist-philosopher René Dubos has pointed out, no society can make a commitment to providing modern medical care to all its citizens who need it without feeling the effects of that commitment in other areas. If modern medical care is provided to everyone, there will be little public money left for other socially valuable programs, in the fields of education, culture, defense, or whatever. Alternatively, as has already begun to happen in Sweden and England, tax rates will be so high that individuals have little money to spend as they choose. Can any society make such sacrifices, even in the name of "health care," and still remain viable and able to grow in other areas?

Another possible course—no less problematical—has been forecast by medical economist Victor Fuchs. Society may have to accept the fact that medical facilities, technologies, personnel, and services will always be in short supply. Choices will then have to be made about which technologies should be developed, and who will have access to scarce medical resources. Who should make such decisions—literally decisions of life and death—and on the basis of what criteria? How should the criteria be established? Such questions already face the committees that must decide which patients will have priority access to life-sustaining therapies like kidney dialysis. The extension to other life and death situations is a logical consequence of adherence to the medical model of health care, unless we are willing to accept the first alternative and curtail personal and public expenditure in other areas.

In addition to the questions of costs and choices, the medical model of health can be challenged in at least one other important area. Medicine as traditionally practiced in the United States has little influence on the familial, job-related, socioeconomic, cultural and other conditions that so frequently lead a person to become a patient. Nor can a person do much about his working and living conditions, however dangerous to his health they may be, unless he has the economic and educational mobility to move or change jobs. Because many of our illnesses and injuries are closely related to the ways we earn, live, and eat, at best medicine deals primarily with symptoms and effects.

Ultimately, the question should be raised as to whether, even with the best of medical care, one can be healthy in a society that itself is unhealthy or fosters ill health or a high risk of injury. Is the health of one who works in a highly competitive or stressful job protected when medicine supplies a chemical agent that helps that person survive? Can a society in which increasing numbers of people turn to addictions and/or crime, while others live in fear of victimi-

zation, be considered healthful? Can many people maintain
a healthful diet in a society whose food processors and
grocers find it most profitable to advertise and sell junk
foods or foods stocked with additives, preservatives, or hormones? The number of questions grow almost daily. Medical ways of responding grow almost as fast, but does that
mean that health care is improving?

Clearly, a serious commitment to health care might
carry us further into questions about our economic and so-
ciocultural institutions than most people want to go, as
those working in the field of public health have long
known. After all, these same institutions are responsible for
the very high standard of living enjoyed by most Americans, even the poorest.

Thus we are brought almost full circle. Substantive interference with these institutions, even in the name of
health, would inevitably involve the infringement of existing rights and changes in established values. The long-term
outcome of substantive change might be a vastly healthier
population. Is this possibility a sufficient base from which
to justify the interference?

Alternative Models

Because of the problems associated with the medical
model of health care, it is important to consider alternatives. The medicine we know today—which regards medicine as an empirical, natural science, considers disease as an
instrumentally verifiable deviation from statistically established norms, and sees human beings in terms of organ systems, biochemical processes, diseases or injuries—is less than
a century old. Moreover, it was established at a time when
it could demonstrate little scientific superiority over available alternatives and it did so in what was largely a political process.

From this follow two questions. It is often asserted or
assumed that the vast array of scientific breakthroughs,
miracle cures and lifesaving technologies of scientific medicine are proof of its superiority to all other approaches to

problems of illness or injury; scientific medicine is even regarded as the *only* valid approach to illness. However, there is room to wonder whether any other approach, if it had enjoyed the "official" status of scientific medicine and the large amounts of public, corporate and private money poured into research based on it, might not have achieved results that were qualitatively as impressive.

The second question is to what extent is it true that scientific medicine "works" for us because, in our scientifically and technologically oriented culture, we *expect* it to work. This is not to suggest that there is no objective foundation to scientific medicine. Nonetheless, most conditions that take people to doctors' offices are conditions that the body itself will eventually heal, or which will result in eventual death regardless of medical interventions. The most medicine does in such cases is to reduce anxiety, pain, and the likelihood of infection, so that the body's self-healing capacities can function unhindered by these secondary conditions. The "primitive" folk healer of China, Ghana, or Bolivia does this no less than the modern European or American physician—and neither group is always successful.

In addition, medical anthropologists are beginning to conclude that the feature most common to all forms of medicine and most crucial in the degree of success achieved is belief. If belief is such a crucial factor in the efficacy of medicine in other cultures, why should scientific medicine be an exception? To be sure, the expectations created by beliefs and the values underlying them vary from culture to culture. But on what grounds could those of one culture be considered more valid than or superior to those of another? Moreover, within our own culture there are documented examples of people who either rejected scientific medicine or whose condition remained unaltered by it, and who have nonetheless experienced apparently miraculous recovery on the basis of belief.

This suggests that considerable insight might be gained from the study of alternatives to scientific medicine. In fact, such work has already begun: conferences, symposia, and workshops have been held over the past few years on such topics as "The Crisis of Values in Science and Medicine," "Health and Healing: Ancient and Modern, Eastern and Western," or "New Boundaries for Health: Self, Family, and Society"; initially under the impetus of the women's movement, publications and efforts are dealing with the various dimensions of self-care; and more and more articles raise critical questions about hospitalization and medicalization. The benefits of childbirth at home or home care for heart attack victims are being studied. The purpose of such exploration is not to eliminate scientific medicine but rather to reconsider the assumption that it represents the only means or always the most appropriate means of health care, and to discover its valid place in the total spectrum of health care. As long as scientific medicine is regarded as the primary factor in health care, rising costs and life-and-death decisions are inevitable.

Thus, ironically, it may be an advantage that the United States is the only advanced country that has not had a national health service or a national health insurance system since the end of World War II. By and large, all countries that have such a service or system are committed institutionally and ideologically to the scientific model of medicine as the means of health care. The results in terms of costs are already evident in England and Sweden, the decision problems are evident in all cases.

The United States is likewise committed to the medical model, but the final decisions regarding how health care will be made a right and financed have not been made. There is still time, in other words, to examine the effects of an uncritical acceptance of the medical model, to consider the legitimate place and role of scientific medicine, and to evaluate alternative models. It is perhaps still possible to establish a flexible system that would permit people to realize their right to health care in ways that correspond to their own needs, beliefs, and conditions, rather than those of the medical professions, the hospitals, and the pharmaceutical and medical equipment industries.

PART TWO: THE SEARCH FOR ANSWERS

V. NATIONAL HEALTH INSURANCE

EDITOR'S INTRODUCTION

Over the past decade, the nation has debated national health insurance (NHI) more or less continuously. Labor unions, church groups, civil rights organizations, and young health professionals have argued for a system that would fulfill what they see as the citizen's right to health care. Private health insurance has failed to provide coverage for nearly 40 million Americans, they point out. For the average subscriber to a private plan, they remind us, insurance covers only 40 percent of all medical-care costs.

The private health-insurance industry has lined up against NHI, as has—until recently—the American Medical Association (AMA). The AMA now backs a bill that would require all employers to offer private insurance plans to their full-time employees.

In 1977, President Jimmy Carter asked the Department of Health, Education, and Welfare to put together a comprehensive national health-insurance plan that could be phased in over a period of four to five years. Yet he soon became convinced that medical-care costs had to be brought under control before any plan could work. The plan that HEW comes up with is expected, for that reason, to be a cautious one, perhaps extending coverage to children and pregnant women before bringing in other segments of the population.

Still, national health insurance seems an idea whose time has come. Leda R. Judd, a former director of national affairs for the National Urban Coalition, makes that clear in this section's first selection, "Federal Involvement in Health Care After 1945," taken from *Current History*. The federal government's role in this area, expanding since World War II, assumed prominence in 1965 with the passage of Medicaid and Medicare. As we move toward some form of national health insurance, the government's considerable influence on the private institutions involved with medical care is sure to become paramount. When—as projected for 1980—nearly 10 percent of the goods and services that the nation produces are related to medical care, the government cannot afford to look the other way. For one thing, the consumers of medical care will not permit it.

The next selection, "Needed: A National Authority," was written by Dr. Charles C. Edwards, a former commissioner of the Food and Drug Administration and assistant secretary of HEW. He recommends running the medical-care system as a public utility, with centralized planning from Washington. The third selection, reprinted from the New York *Times Magazine*, is written by Richard J. Margolis, freelance writer, who maintains that since every other industrialized country in the world provides its citizens with some form of national health insurance or direct medical care through a national health service, the United States is, in a way, a holdout.

Can the nation afford NHI? Not unless the plan keeps costs down, says Harvard Professor Martin Feldstein, in this section's fourth excerpt. His proposal, "Major-Risk Insurance," ties NHI to a schedule of copayments based on the citizen's ability to pay so that the consumer of medical services would share the costs with the government—and have a stake in keeping those costs low.

The final piece in this section is an interview with Dr. Richard Palmer, president of the American Medical Association in 1976, by a staff member of the *National Observer*. Dr. Palmer makes the case for the Carter-Hansen bill, which the AMA supports, and for keeping the federal government and the practice of medicine as separate as possible.

FEDERAL INVOLVEMENT IN HEALTH CARE AFTER 1945 [1]

As spending on health has mushroomed, so has the role of the federal government, not only in paying for care but in the area of deciding how and where care would be delivered. In 1929, public expenditures accounted for 13.3 percent of the total expenditures on health. By 1950, the percentage had increased to 19.1 percent and by 1975 it had grown to 42.2 percent....

The bulk of the federal health dollar (69 percent) finances or directly provides health care services (14 percent). Most of the remainder supports the development of health resources through research (7 percent), manpower training (4 percent) or facilities construction (3 percent).

The federal involvement in health began its expansion following World War II, and the growth rate accelerated with the passage of Medicare and Medicaid in 1965. Initially, federal involvement included paying for research, the construction of facilities and the education of health professionals. With the coming of the "War on Poverty" in the 1960s and the passage of Medicare and Medicaid, a federal role in both delivery of care and payment for care was created.

The government's involvement can be divided into seven broad general categories that cover most of its health activities: health research; health manpower training; construction of health facilities; prevention and control of health problems; provision of health services and the financing of care. The seventh and most recent area of federal involvement is the attempt at regulation of the health-care field with primary emphasis on cost control. Regulation, of course, has an impact on each of the other areas of federal involvement.

[1] From article by Leda R. Judd, former director of national affairs, National Urban Coalition. *Current History.* 72:201–6+. My./Je. '77. Copyright © 1977 by Current History, Inc. Reprinted by permission.

Health Research

The federal government has been involved in health research since 1878, when it created the United States Public Health Service and assigned it the task of investigating the causes and control of epidemics.

After World War II, expenditures for medical research from all sources expanded from 2 cents per capita in 1940 to $12.50 in 1974. The federal government's share of these expenditures has grown to more than 60 percent. Some of this research is being carried out by the National Institutes of Health and related federal facilities, but most research is done at medical schools and hospitals under federal grant and contract arrangements. This aspect of federal "involvement" in health care has met with almost no opposition from organized medicine. . . .

Estimates are that federal expenditures for health-related research will total just over $3 billion in fiscal year 1977, an increase from the $2.8 billion spent in 1976 and the $2.8 billion and $2.5 billion outlays for 1974 and 1975. While overall funds for health research are growing, health research investment is declining as a percentage of total health expenditures. Many research projects now sponsored by the government are directed toward specific disease categories such as cancer. . . .

Health Manpower Training

A student entering Georgetown University Medical School in Washington, D.C., in 1977 will pay a first year's *tuition* of more than $10,000. According to the university, this increase from $6,800 in 1976 (and $5,000 in 1975) is necessary because of a 1976 federal law redirecting funds available to medical schools for medical education. Before the passage of this 1976 law, the Health Professions Assistance Act, it is estimated that the federal government was paying 60 percent of the cost of each physician's education.

The government has traditionally been involved in providing training programs for personnel in Veterans Administration and Defense Department facilities. After World War II, the federal government made an effort to upgrade and improve the quality of care provided by the Veterans Administration (VA) hospitals. The affiliation of these hospitals with medical schools was authorized by Congress in 1946; by 1974, 116 VA hospitals had established these affiliations. . . .

Beginning in the late 1950s, the government began to play additional roles in the financing of medical education. In addition to the monies from research grants that were an indirect means of financing medical schools, a series of direct federal financing programs for medical education were enacted.

☐ In 1956, funds were authorized for traineeships for public health personnel and for advanced training for nurses.

☐ In 1958, formula grants were authorized for schools of public health.

☐ In 1963, a major program of institutional grants designed to remedy a shortage of health professionals was enacted. These grants were contingent on increased first-year enrollments and provided funds for construction or improvement of medical school facilities and a variety of special projects. Over the years, these grants grew until they included not only physicians, nurses and dentists, but pharmacists, podiatrists, veterinarians, allied health professionals and schools of public health.

☐ In 1971, these grants were replaced by a new system of grants based upon a payment for each student enrolled (capitation payment), contingent upon increased first-year enrollments. Start-up assistance to new schools was also provided.

As a result of this series of federal programs, by 1974 the government was largely responsible for the building of twenty-one medical schools, nine dental schools and a school of osteopathic medicine. Medical schools increased the size of their entering classes from 8,298 students in 1960–1961 to 14,963 in 1974, an 80 percent increase.

Increasing enrollments in health-professions schools created a new problem—how to finance the cost of education for many of the students. Beginning in 1963, a series of federal loan and scholarship programs was enacted. These programs not only provided funds to students but, using loan forgiveness and scholarship provisions, gave the federal government some leverage with which to encourage students to practice in areas that lacked an adequate supply of health personnel or in areas of specialization that had been neglected. Congress also created a National Health Service Corps to encourage physicians to practice in isolated, doctor-short areas of the country. Students who joined the corps would receive ample scholarships in exchange for a commitment to practice for a specified period in an underserved area. In 1975, there were 551 health professionals in 268 communities throughout the country.

It was hoped, of course, that once physicians were situated in these areas they would remain, thus easing the shortage and rectifying the severe maldistribution of health resources in this country. This does not seem to have occurred. Geographic maldistribution of health personnel and resources remains one of the serious unsolved problems of the health-care system.

The newly enacted Health Professions Assistance Act attempts to use federal funds to remedy this problem. Authorization of funds for the National Health Service Corps will be enlarged; medical schools are required to train specified numbers of residents in primary care in order to obtain funds; student loan and loan repayment programs are to be more restrictive unless students agree to practice in shortage areas; more scholarships are to be provided to needy students; and restrictions will be tightened on the entry of foreign medical graduates. No federal manpower program has yet had any significant impact on where physicians chose to practice; and it remains to be seen if this one will.

Construction of Health Facilities

In addition to contributing a large share of the monies needed to build medical and other professional schools, the federal government also has paid out more than $5 billion in grants and loans to build hospitals. This money was channeled through the Hospital Survey and Construction Act of 1946 (the Hill-Burton act). Hill-Burton provided the necessary financial impetus for the rapid growth of hospitals.

During the depression of the 1930s and World War II, hospital construction came to a halt. Hill-Burton was enacted to remedy what was considered to be a shortage of hospital beds—particularly in smaller towns and cities. Subsequent amendments authorized grants for the construction of other types of health facilities and for the replacement of obsolete facilities, with a priority for requests from urban areas. Recent years have seen a shift from direct grant funds to loans and loan guarantees, and from the construction of new hospitals to the modernization or addition of services like outpatient clinics to existing facilities.

It is generally agreed that there is no longer a shortage of hospital beds. Indeed, it is claimed that we are oversupplied. The federal share of national expenditures for health facilities construction dropped by about 30 percent between 1965 and 1975.

During its twenty-nine-year history, the Hill-Burton program appropriated and spent over $4.1 billion in grant funds for construction or modernization; more than $1 billion in loan principal (either direct or guaranteed) was also committed. A total of 11,493 grant projects were approved, accounting for nearly 496,000 beds in hospitals and long-term-care facilities, as well as 3,450 outpatient and other health-care facilities. More than 3,969 communities have been aided in the construction or modernization of 6,549 public and nonprofit facilities.

Of the $14.5 billion which these projects cost, the Hill-Burton share was $4.1 billion, 28 percent of the total. The other $10.4 billion came from state and local sources. Without Hill-Burton funds as seed money, many of these projects would not have been initiated. Hill-Burton was successful in increasing not only the supply but also the quality of health-care facilities. The very success of the program, however, is now creating problems since the existence of all these facilities contributes to the bias of the United States health-care system in favor of in-hospital care. Often this bias operates at the expense of the development of less costly alternative modes of care. . . .

Prevention and Control of Health Problems

As costs of health care escalate, so do the cries that if we spent more on preventive care, we would spend less on sickness care—and prevention is cheaper. Many federal agencies are involved in the prevention and control of health problems. Yet exclusive of the work of the Environmental Protection Agency all these efforts amount to only approximately 3 or 4 percent of all federal expenditures for health. In 1976, the federal government reported approximately $1.3 billion in expenditures for all disease prevention, environmental control and consumer protection programs.

From the National Center for Disease Control established in 1946 to the new National Center for Health Education established in 1976, a myriad of federal organizations have worked on pieces of the prevention problem. Agencies whose functions are directly related to the prevention of disease and ill health and the maintenance of a healthy population include the Occupational Safety and Health Administration in the Department of Labor, the Food and Drug Administration, and the Environmental Protection Agency.

All these agencies have been accused of inadequately protecting the nation's health. They, in turn, have charged that they are underfunded and understaffed and that many of their goals can only be reached by improving American "health habits" and awareness. . . .

The Provision of Health Services

The federal government "provides" health services to certain populations directly through programs like the clinics and hospitals that served Armed Forces personnel and their families and the extensive network of veterans (VA) hospitals. Disabled seamen, Indians, and federal prisoners also are direct recipients of federal care. Of the total federal health expenditures in 1974, about 8 percent went for Defense Department health facilities and another 8 percent for VA facilities.

The government also provides care indirectly through grants to state and local governments, institutions and organizations to provide services to particular populations. Generally, these programs serve needy persons. Most of these programs have been established since World War II and grew out of the government's concern over the inadequacy of services available to certain groups at risk in our society —children, the disabled, the poor.

Among these programs are maternal and child health programs that provide health services for pregnant women, infants, and children with certain handicapping conditions (services are provided primarily in rural and economically depressed areas); rehabilitation programs providing support for state and local programs for treatment of disabilities from diseases like epilepsy, stroke, and cerebral palsy; family planning programs; alcohol and narcotic treatment programs; programs and facilities for the mentally retarded; community Mental Health Centers that serve approximately one million people per year; programs to develop and improve emergency medical services on an areawide basis.

One of the most effective government programs has been the financing of neighborhood health centers, and migrant health centers. Initially established by the Migrant Health Act of 1962 and the Economic Opportunity Act of 1964, approximately 160 of these centers serve almost 2 million people across the country.

In 1976, the total outlay for all these programs, including the National Health Service Corps, which is included with these programs for budget purposes (and some other smaller programs) totaled about $1.1 billion—less than 3 percent of the total federal health budget.

These programs have brought quality care to people who need it, but they have only filled in gaps—they have not made any significant impact on the organization and basic health-care delivery system in this country. People who can pay and who have private health insurance generally use a private physician; those who cannot pay often rely on federal programs. These programs have been criticized as perpetuating a "two-class" medical care system, with those who can pay receiving one kind of care, and those who cannot, a lesser quality of care.

Nonetheless, the federal government will probably continue to support these programs and encourage their development as models of how care could be delivered to a larger public.

Financing Care

These federal programs account for less than one half of the federal expenditure for health. The largest federal health programs, in terms of dollars and impact, have been Medicare and Medicaid, which in 1976 accounted for more than 70 percent of all federal health-care spending.

By terms of the Social Security Amendments of 1965, Medicare and Medicaid established a major role for the federal government in financing health care. The government had enacted several minor programs as forerunners, particularly the 1960 Kerr-Mills act, which authorized federal/state cost-sharing for the health needs of certain aged persons. But these early efforts at providing care for the aged and poor amounted to only about $550 million.

Briefly, Medicare, Title 18 of the Social Security Act, provides health insurance to persons aged sixty-five and over who are eligible for Social Security. Medicaid, Title 19, is a federally assisted state program that offers health benefits to low-income individuals on public assistance and, in some states, to those regarded as "medically needy" because their incomes are only slightly higher than welfare standards. Depending on the per capita income of a state's population, the federal government pays between 50 and 78 percent of the costs of a state's Medicaid program. Within broad federal guidelines, the states, determine the eligibility of recipients, the scope of services provided, and the amounts paid to providers.

The Medicare and Medicaid programs have grown so rapidly that in 1975 they accounted for more than $27.7 billion in health spending. . . .

These programs have come under increasing fire. Allegations of scandal, particularly in the Medicaid program, of mismanagement, of fraud and abuse by providers, appear almost daily, tending to obscure the programs' tangible benefits to the aged and the poor. . . .

What are the lessons of Medicare and Medicaid? Clearly, enacting a new federal program and providing more dollars will probably not bring order to the chaotic health-care delivery system in the United States.

The inequities in the availability, quality and cost of care have led the federal government increasingly into the area of regulation of the health-care field. Laws aimed at cost, utilization and quality control are already using the federal dollar as a lever. None of them have been particularly successful.

Experimental health-delivery programs, like the Health Maintenance Organization Act of 1973 that sought to stimulate prepaid group practices providing comprehensive care to members for a fixed fee, have encountered the resistance of organized medicine and the disinterest of the public at large. [See "Containing the Cost of Employee Health Plans," in Section VI, below.]

The federal government has also enacted health planning laws to try to assure the orderly development and use of resources. The National Health Planning and Resources Development Act of 1974 is potentially the most far-reaching of the planning measures, in terms of expanded government regulation of the health-care delivery system. The 1974 act mandates a far more comprehensive planning program than its predecessors. The network of state and area planning agencies provided for in the act has wide responsibilities, including the development and implementation of a state-wide services and facilities plan, and review of the appropriateness of existing institutional services and facilities and proposals for expansion. It is too early to judge the impact of this program.

In the area of cost control pressures for regulation are mounting, and in this area there is relatively little that the federal government can do short of actual wage and price controls. There are proposals to limit hospital costs by requiring hospitals to set budget limits each year through negotiation with the government. The government's lever would, of course, be the share of costs paid through Medicare and Medicaid. Physicians, nursing homes, laboratory testing and other segments of the industry that have contributed to inflationary pressures are even more difficult to control.

Today, the federal government must try to find an effective new way to attack the health-care problem, which has frustrated the government for years and shows no signs of going away.

NEEDED: A NATIONAL AUTHORITY [2]

It only seems fair to assert that the economic plight of the American health-care system reflects a serious failure of leadership within the health establishment. The private sector has made regrettably little effort either to address the causes of the economic crisis or to work with public agencies toward their solution.

But the record of public leadership is not notably more illustrious or successful. Federal health officials have tried

[2] Article entitled "Rx for Health Care—a National Authority," by Dr. Charles C. Edwards, former commissioner of the U.S. Food and Drug Administration, now senior vice president of a medical instrumentation firm. Washington *Post*. p C 1. Mr. 7. '76. Copyright © 1976, Field Enterprises Inc., reproduced through the courtesy of Field Newspaper Syndicate.

to develop and articulate a national health strategy, but the government's fiscal managers have been little inclined to go along with such planning. Instead, they have come up with schemes that offer nothing more than reduced federal spending by means of the dubious expedient of turning major health-service programs over to the states; most of the states cannot afford to run such programs and certainly are less able than the national government to bring about fundamental change.

The fiscal managers' zeal is prompted by the hard fact that federal health spending, especially for Medicare and Medicaid, has skyrocketed in recent years. Unfortunately, however, the budgetary remedy they propose will do virtually nothing to control costs, to improve the quality of care or to reform the system itself. In the absence of effective leadership in either the private or the public-health sector, the prospect for needed change seems remote at best.

What remedy is there? If the present track seems to be leading to disaster, how do we get off it and what other track do we seek? Is there the basis for reform in a closely controlled system of national health insurance? And if so, how do we go about it?

Beyond any question, present systems of health insurance have contributed to the economic crisis. But it *is* possible that a national financing system, properly designed and managed, could become as potent a remedy as present systems have been potent problems. And perhaps the first step toward this transformation is to treat the pluralistic health-care system as a public utility rather than as an overgrown cottage industry, a political football, a subset of the welfare state or any of a number of other interpretations that fit the narrow viewpoints of special interests as diverse as the American Medical Association and the United Auto Workers.

The Public Utility Model

The public utility model would seem to be justified on a number of grounds. For one, health care is an essential public service, albeit a service that is provided largely through private enterprise. Further, there is virtually no inherent competition in the health-care system. A patient may choose this or that physician as a matter of personal preference or informed judgment, but the patient cannot, in any practical sense, compare one provider with another. Even the choice of physician or insurance plan has little effect on the way the health-care system will perform or on the cost of services. Finally, the health-care system is heavily supported by public expenditures. Fifty percent of the cost of physician education, the vast majority of the cost of research and about a third of the cost of health care are paid for through taxes. Thus, the concept of the health-care system as a public utility is neither illogical nor inappropriate. On the contrary, it amounts to a frank recognition of the status quo as the starting point for necessary change.

Managed as a public utility, the health-care system would be subject to public regulation to make sure that its day-to-day activities and its long-range plans were consistent with a realistic and on-going assessment of public needs. Under such a concept, national health insurance would be not merely a means of softening the economic burden without really doing anything to reduce it, but a tangible instrument—one of several—to make the health-care system fully accountable and fully responsible to the public served.

But if a public utility model is to work, it will have to have at its head a national health authority empowered to control the economics of the system, to determine how its resources—both public and private—are allocated and to decide what measures and changes are needed to assure quality and adequacy of care.

A national health authority, generally analogous to the Federal Reserve Board, would have to be granted broad powers by the Congress: the power to establish rates and fee schedules on a regional basis, to approve or reject construction plans, to determine manpower requirements and see that they are met, to regulate public and private health-insurance plans, to establish national licensing and certification procedures for health professionals and allied health workers, to advise the President and the Congress on legislative and budgetary matters and have its advice treated as authoritative, if not binding.

In essence, the authority would function as a national board of health, free of political constraint, free of professional or institutional bias and armed with sufficient regulatory powers and the sanctions to make its decisions stick.

Appointed by the President and subject to Senate confirmation, the members of a national health authority would have to be broadly representative of medicine and other health professions, hospitals, the scientific-academic community, the insurance industry and consumers. Members should serve for terms of at least six years in order to keep partisan politics out of both the selection of members and the judgments and decisions of the national health authority.

It is abundantly clear that health policy has become a major political issue over the last two decades, a state of affairs that has frustrated efforts at rational planning and sound management. At a very minimum, a national health authority could serve to turn this around, to put the urgent and continuing business of leadership in competent hands and divorce it from partisan politics.

Time Running Out

Any proposal to create a powerful governing body for the American health-care system will surely be anathema to a great many individuals and organizations. Organized medicine strenuously opposes virtually any hint of regulation and has, in fact, gone to court to block a program of peer review that would require doctors to monitor their own performance in treating Medicare patients. And in a larger sense, at a time of strong opposition to federal regulation of the marketplace, the suggestion that the American health-care system needs more rather than less governmental control will seem out of step with both political and ideological trends.

But what is the alternative? The alternative is further unrestrained escalation in the cost of care, more ill-conceived legislation enacted on a piecemeal basis to serve short-term political goals and, ultimately, the irresistible demand for nationalization of a system that lacks the ability to control itself in the public interest, to say nothing of its own.

At this late hour, with time running out, a national health authority is the only workable alternative to total collapse of a system that cannot survive without responsible public regulation.

THE DREAM WHOSE TIME HAS COME? [3]

The history of national health insurance in this country is strewn with predictions about its imminent arrival.

Part of the trouble may arise from the complexity of our burgeoning medical system, which defies instant rehabilitation, and from the apparently high price we must pay for its reform. Many of the recently tried solutions, notably Medicare and Medicaid, have themselves become part of the problem, encouraging waste and driving up costs. . . .

The new Congress and the new President will have to confront this general paradox of social progress, in which measures designed to lighten the burden of some may end by increasing the burden of all. . . .

Franklin D. Roosevelt came within an ace of combining health insurance with Social Security in 1935, only to be dissuaded by the AMA [American Medical Association], notably by Dr. Harvey Cushing, author, brain surgeon and father-in-law of young James Roosevelt.

Whatever recommendations F.D.R. might decide to make, Cushing wrote to the President, "no legislation can

[3] Excerpts from "National Health Insurance—the Dream Whose Time Has Come?" by Richard J. Margolis, freelance writer. New York *Times Magazine*. p 12–13+. Ja. 9, '77. © 1977 by The New York Times Company. Reprinted by permission.

be effective without the good will of the American Medical Association, which has the organization to put it to work." In the politics of health reform, Cushing's comment remains the heart of the matter; and nowadays politicians must seek the cooperation not only of the AMA but also of other health interest-groups that have grown up in the interim. Over the decades our health-care system has invented a potpourri of patchwork schemes as substitutes for "the lost reform," and each new expedient—Blue Cross, for example, in the thirties and forties—has given rise to a new organization in Washington. Like all newcomers, these organizations have become instantly suspicious of change and broadly committed to things as they are. If Cushing were alive today, he could cite at least four other groups whose good will may now be required: the "Blues," the private insurance industry, the hospitals and the medical schools.

The battle did not end with the New Deal. Harry S. Truman took up the cudgels, to secure passage of the Murray-Wagner-Dingell bill, a measure the AMA dismissed as "Marxist medicine." It never reached the floor of Congress, but it has since seen several reincarnations.

Considering the discouraging record, it wasn't any wonder that both John F. Kennedy and Lyndon B. Johnson chose to fight on narrower ground. Each came to the White House prepared to settle for something less than "the lost reform." With the passage of Medicare and Medicaid in 1965, the Congress conferred the blessings of free or low-cost medical care upon both the elderly and the poor. The new programs enlarged the public's sense of possibilities. . . .

The Congress began to consider new measures, a fresh generation of legislative proposals that would extend the protection of health insurance to some or all of the remaining population. Such proposals have grown more numerous of late. . . . [In the Ninety-fourth Congress] no less than eighteen different bills were submitted, each alleging to offer the most practical solutions. These plans are Jimmy Carter's health-reform legacy.

If the titles sound maddeningly alike, their contents exhibit some real differences. By and large, they reflect the contradictory hopes of people and organizations who have something to gain or lose from the redistribution of health care in America—doctors, hospitals, insurers, medical schools and patients. As consumers and taxpayers, one can try to test the merits of the proposals by keeping close to two familiar touchstones: the benefits offered and the costs incurred. In addition, one can examine any bill for its reform potential, meaning the extent to which it can be expected to reorganize health care along lines that make sense.

Of the eighteen now before Congress a half dozen perhaps can be considered "major," either because of the power and celebrity of their congressional sponsors or because of the influence of their outside backers. Like the lobbies that support them, these six are a mixed bag. All but one would make health insurance compulsory. They range from a modest proposal that would extend benefits to citizens who have incurred unusually high medical costs—the so-called "Catastrophic Health Insurance and Medical Assistance Reform Act," introduced by Democratic Senators Russell Long of Louisiana and Abraham Ribicoff of Connecticut—to the sweeping "Health Security" measure that Senator Edward M. Kennedy [Democrat, Massachusetts] has been promoting since 1969. . . .

Besides Kennedy-Corman and Long-Ribicoff, four proposals seem worth considering, listed here in a sequence that runs from the relatively broad and generous to the relatively narrow and penny-pinching:

☐ The "Comprehensive Health Insurance Plan" (CHIP), introduced by Kentucky Democratic Representative Lee Carter—no relation. It has been called a "block off the old CHIP" because it closely resembles a bill of the same name that the Nixon Administration submitted to the Congress in 1973. A nearly identical plan, moreover, in

1974 almost got past Wilbur Mills's House Ways and Means Committee, the historic gatekeeper of health reform. [See "AMA President Discusses Health Care Costs," below in this section.]

☐ A complex proposal submitted by Representative Al Ullman, an Oregon Democrat, who succeeded Mills as Ways and Means chairman; it is called the "National Health Care Services Reorganization and Financing Act," quite a mouthful, and it has the official blessings of the American Hospital Association.

☐ The AMA's latest entry, "The Comprehensive Health Care Insurance Act," sponsored by Representative Richard Fulton, a Tennessee Democrat.

☐ And "The National Health Care Act," a favorite of the Health Insurance Association of America (HIAA). It was introduced by two conservative Democrats, Senator Thomas McIntyre of New Hampshire and Representative Omar Burleson of Texas.

As might be expected, not all of the bills confront all of the problems; by and large they concentrate on ways of defraying patient costs and of spreading patient benefits, with the unspoken hope that the rest will take care of itself. Still, with the exception of Long-Ribicoff—which continues Medicare's blank-check system of reimbursement—the proposals do make an effort to curb inflation. The chief restraining device envisioned in these bills entails an annual round of negotiations, with doctors and hospitals, on all fees and rates; an attempt to commit the health-care industry each year to an immutable schedule of charges. In all but the Kennedy-Corman measure, the responsibility for negotiating these schedules is assigned to the individual states; only Kennedy-Corman, which we shall consider first, sees the federal government as prime negotiator.

The Kennedy-Corman Health Security bill calls for a compulsory federalized system of health care managed within HEW [the Department of Health, Education, and

Welfare] by a five-member health-security board, and financed chieflly through a half-and-half combination of payroll taxes and general revenues. As is the case with most of the other bills, the payroll taxes are shared by employers and employees. The benefits offered by Kennedy-Corman are broad, generous and virtually free of the kinds of restrictions one finds in the other proposals. But the benefits are not the whole story; what distinguishes this bill from all others is its unique approach to budgeting, an approach that makes private enterprise an instrument of public policy.

Health Security stops short of nationalizing the health-care system, but it does nationalize the health-care budget. Every dollar spent—whether for construction of a new hospital or for purchase of a new tongue depressor—becomes a federal dollar. The budgeting process is supposed to begin at the local levels where groups of consumers and professionals annually assess their health-care needs and estimate the costs. These estimates filter up through a regionalized system and eventually land in Washington on the health-security board's desk, becoming part of the year's national health-care budget.

Cost controls under Kennedy-Corman turn traditional procedures upside-down: The bill stipulates that the annual health-care budget cannot exceed expected revenues, thereby tying the medical budget to the fortunes of the general economy. If the economy should slip, the federal government would have to negotiate a reduced budget, and the bill's supporters insist that the burden of such a reduction would be assumed not by the patient but by the health-care providers. In other words, rather than curtailing services, Kennedy-Corman would curtail the fees and rates paid to doctors and hospitals. The proposal thus jeopardizes the industry's time-honored privilege of controlling fees and services, one reason for the measure's bad reputation among medical practitioners. On the other hand, it enjoys sustained support from both the AFL-CIO and the United Auto

Workers, as well as from a coalition of church groups and liberal-leaning organizations like Common Cause and the Urban League. It is the only proposal thus far to have attracted substantial consumer backing. [For a brief statement of the AMA view of this legislation see "AMA President Discusses Health-Care Costs," below, in this Section.]

The Long-Ribicoff proposal is a "major-medical" plan to insure patients against costly illness. Its benefits, presumably, begin about the time a patient has run out of money: after he has spent two thousand dollars for medical services or has been in the hospital for sixty days. An employer can buy this insurance for his employee either from the government, in which case he pays a 1 percent payroll tax, or he can choose a government-approved private plan—Blue Cross, for instance. (As with nearly all the bills, this one makes special provision for both the self-employed and the poor.)

Compared with Kennedy's Health Security proposal, Long-Ribicoff seems both paltry and narrow. It leaves the gears and levers of the health-care enterprise untouched, and the benefits it provides, while they may save some families from bankruptcy, are far from dazzling. Still, the measure has a certain appeal. It is simple and can be immediately "put into place," as the health analysts like to say, whereas most of the other plans would take years to become fully effective. It is also inexpensive, at least from the standpoint of federal budgeting; and it can be seen not as the Grand Solution but as merely a first step toward eventual enactment of "the lost reform."

Finally, the bill gives the health-insurance industry a piece of the action, an idea that may or may not have merit, but which in any case can be seen to make some tactical sense. It will come as no surprise that the private insurance companies are said to have bestowed their tacit approval upon this modest measure—in fact, to have taken a hand in its drafting. A Kennedy-Corman aficionado claims last year [1976] to have seen "at least a dozen of the insurance boys

from Hartford in the back of the hearing room, just before
the hearing started, making last-minute changes in the bill."
The Ribicoff aides I have talked to say this is news to them;
but it is true that an earlier version of the Long-Ribicoff
bill provided for *federal insurance only*, leaving no room
for participation by private companies.

In any event, because Senator Long is chairman of the
Finance Committee, the womb from which any successful
Senate bill must issue, the proposal has not lacked for a
public platform.

Nor has CHIP, the Nixon bill that never dies. Benefits
under CHIP are in some respects as far-reaching as those
under Kennedy-Corman, but they include a $150 deductible
for each person and also a 25 percent "coinsurance" requirement; that is, the family must pay either one fourth of its
health-care charges or $1,500, whichever is less during a
given year. All this is to be financed not by taxes but by
premiums paid directly to private insurance companies by
employees and their employers; the latter group pays the
larger share.

Unlike the other two bills, CHIP leaves virtually all of
the program's management to insurance firms and to the
individual states, with the federal government playing a
small, regulatory role. Each state makes its own reimbursement policy, deciding how much money doctors and other
providers should be paid for their services. The formula is
similar to that now being used under Medicaid, and given
that program's record, it is not a promising one. Nevertheless, CHIP has impressed some Congressmen as a workable
compromise between "the two extremes" of catastrophic insurance and Health Security. It offers citizens more than the
first and it costs the government less than the second.

The remaining three proposals, like CHIP, give citizens
a chance to buy private health-insurance at modest cost,
entitling them to a variety of benefits, but the benefits are
hedged with coinsurance charges and other limits, and they,
too, are essentially devoid of cost controls, with all administrative responsibility ceded to the states. What makes these

proposals interesting is not the substance of their ideas but the nature of their support. Each is officially backed by a different lobby, and each can tell us something about the aspirations of the health-care network.

Al Ullman's bill, backed by the American Hospital Association, may be the most Byzantine. Besides the insurance and financing provisions, the act mandates creation in every locale of health-care corporations to which citizens may subscribe in advance of services. Apparently, these corporations would function as health maintenance organizations (HMOs), which is what medical commentators now call groups that offer services on a prepaid basis. The doctors working for HMOs earn salaries or else are paid capitation fees—so much per member-patient. Either way, they are cut loose from standard fee-for-service arrangements and thus from temptations to overcharge or overtreat. Studies have shown that in HMOs the incidence of needless surgery is far less than it is in fee-for-service practice. [For additional information on HMOs see Section VI below.]

All of which sounds promising—but it is not clear from the bill how these local health-care corporations would operate or whether, in fact, an employer or employee could not skirt the corporation entirely and buy his health care from other sources. What does seem clear is that hospitals would play a central role in the new system, since in most places they are the only institutions extant that are capable of developing and managing so complex a plan.

The AMA's bill is less generous than CHIP and less ambitious than Ullman's. It would leave fee-for-service practice and private-insurance precedents unscathed, with the federal government content to mandate the size of the premiums the subscribers would pay and to let the system lurch ahead on its own. To the self-employed wishing to buy insurance, the bill offers a few tax advantages; to the poor it provides "subsidy certificates" they can cash in at their local insurance company. As inadequate as this seems, its represents the farthest AMA members have yet traveled down the road to "Marxist medicine." An earlier, and less-liberal, AMA-backed measure, Medicredit, had to be discarded after the post-Watergate elections of 1974, when fifty-five of its Congressional sponsors were defeated. (The AFL-CIO ran a nationwide campaign to unseat these enemies of Health Security, using the slogan "Your Congressman may be dangerous to your health.")

Finally, there is the "National Health-Care Act," the darling of the HIAA. It has the distinction of being the only plan among the six that permits employers to dismiss it—which is to say that the program is strictly voluntary. If an employer chooses not to buy in, his employees are out of luck. In consequence, the bill has been given short shrift everywhere but in the executive suites of insurance companies. As a labor lobbyist remarked recently, "When you get a proposal that offers less than the AMA does, what have you got? . . . Nothing."

We can pay our money, then, and take our choice, though it is not at all certain just how much money we shall have to pay. A recent HEW study indicates that all six programs are costly—some are more costly than others, but the differences may not be all that great.

The man who conducted the study is Gordon R. Trapnell, a consulting actuary. According to Trapnell, if we enact no new health-care programs during the rest of the decade and continue spending at the present rate, medical costs will rise to $180.2 billion by 1980—a gain of about 30 percent over this year's tab. From that empyrean base, Trapnell calculated the additional costs that might be incurred by each of the six plans, concluding that the three cheapest were Long-Ribicoff, CHIP and the HIAA's voluntary plan. Each would cost at least an extra $10 billion annually. The other three proposals would each run more than twice that amount—an additional $20 billion in the case of the AMA's program, and an extra $25 billion for Ullman or Kennedy-Corman.

Trapnell's estimates suggest that health-care inflation will remain part of the picture regardless of which program the Congress enacts. Any new plan, he notes, will increase administrative expenses and encourage wider use of medical services, especially among the poor. Yet supporters of Kennedy-Corman continue to insist that their proposal is more or less inflation-proof—in part, because it subsidizes *preventive* medicine and, in part, because its budget is linked to national productivity. "We have the only measure with built-in controls," says Max Fine, who directs the Committee for National Health Insurance, a labor-financed lobby.

Many remain skeptical, among them HEW's Saul Waldman, whose detailed 210-page summary of all eighteen health-insurance bills is the bible of analysts and lobbyists alike. "Nobody really knows whether Health Security could keep the lid on," he says. "True, there's a ceiling on the budget, but there's also a clause in the bill that says Congress can be asked for supplemental funds in case of emergencies. The emergency wouldn't necessarily have to be medical, like an epidemic; it could be an *economic* emergency."

On balance, though, the Kennedy-Corman bill does appear to encourage a fiscal climate in which health-care prices will rise no faster than prices overall. The probability under Kennedy-Corman is one of controlled inflation, something we haven't seen in health-care circles since the Nixon price freeze; it would amount to a mild revolution within the health-care industry—a revolution of reimbursements.

But the revolution that Health Security invites us all to join goes beyond fiscal policy. At bottom, it represents a major shift of power and responsibility within the health-care network, a shift away from state governments and private insurance companies toward HEW and the federal bureaucracy. All other plans cede administrative control to the states (under federal guidelines) and commercial control to the private insurers. In opposing Kennedy-Corman, the health-insurance industry is fighting for its very existence. The stakes are high. Last year the industry collected nearly $30 billion in premiums.

MAJOR-RISK INSURANCE [4]

Several years ago, I outlined an approach to national health insurance that I still believe can serve these two objectives. The basic idea in this proposal is extremely simple: Provide every family with an insurance policy so that a family's spending on health care need never be more than a moderate fraction of its income—*but* use a system of copayments to make most families conscious of the cost of their use of health-care services. In the next few pages I will summarize the form of such a national health insurance plan. But it will help to focus and clarify the discussion if I indicate at the outset the six objectives by which we should judge any proposed system of financing health care:

1. *It should prevent deprivation of care.* No one should go without medical care because of inability to pay.

2. *It should prevent financial hardship.* No family should suffer substantial financial hardship because of the expense of unforeseen illness or accident.

3. *It should keep costs down.* A financing system should both encourage efficient use of resources and discourage medical-care price inflation. Whenever possible, patients should use relatively low-cost ambulatory facilities rather than high-cost in-hospital care. Hospitals should be induced to moderate the forces that raise the cost of care: increased personnel, unnecessary pay raises, and a proliferation of technical facilities and services. Physicians should not be encouraged to increase their fees by the knowledge that, because of insurance, the cost to their own patients will rise little, if at all. In short, the financing method should encourage cost-consciousness in the decisions of patients, doctors, and hospital administrators.

4. *It should avoid a large tax increase.* A national health insurance program that raises substantial funds from tax-

[4] From "The High Cost of Hospitals and What to Do About It?" by Martin Feldstein, author, educator, Harvard professor, president of National Bureau of Economic Research. *Public Interest.* 48:49–54. Summer '77. Copyright 1977 by National Affairs, Inc. Reprinted by permission.

payers and returns it in the form of health insurance has a large hidden cost. By reducing the incentive to work, to invest, and to take economic risks, the increased tax rates would lower real national income. The magnitude of our total spending on health care makes this an important consideration. In fiscal year 1976, private health-care expenditures approached $78 billion; transferring this private spending to the public sector would require a very large increase in tax rates.

5. *It should be easily administered.* The administration of a health-care system should not require complex procedures that are costly and inconvenient, or permit arbitrary decisions that will be resented.

6. *It should be generally acceptable.* Any new method of financing should be acceptable to physicians and hospitals, as well as the general public. A system that is disliked by any of these would encounter substantial political opposition and, if instituted, would be hampered by a lack of cooperation.

Before looking at the possible alternatives, let us examine the existing system. Although almost every American is now covered by some form of private or public insurance, the current coverage is still often surprisingly "shallow." That is, families incurring huge medical bills too often find that their insurance pays only a relatively small portion of them. A 1970 National Opinion Research Survey, updated to 1976 prices, found that more than 500,000 families had *out-of-pocket* expenditures of more than $3,000 for medical care. More than two million families spent over $1,500, and more than 10 percent of all families spent over $1,200 out-of-pocket. Let me repeat: These expenses are out-of-pocket, i.e., *after* private and public insurance payments and reimbursements.

Although hospital insurance pays a high proportion of hospital bills, current policies generally impose a variety of ceilings on the use of benefits. The absence of "deep" coverage leaves a serious residue of financial hardship and also prevents some people from seeking potentially expensive care. We have already seen how the current system of financing medical care has contributed to the rapidly rising cost of care. In short, the current structure of health insurance fails by each of the first three criteria that I have suggested.

Uniform Comprehensive Health Insurance

The most widely debated proposals for national health insurance call for a program of universal, uniform, and comprehensive health insurance, something like an extension of Medicare to the entire population. The most comprehensive of these proposals, such as the Kennedy-Corman bill, would even abolish the small deductible and coinsurance provisions of Medicare, eliminate any limit on the length of covered hospitalization, and extend coverage to drugs, dental care, and even housekeeping services.

There is no doubt that under comprehensive insurance no one would be deprived of needed care because of inability to pay, or would suffer any financial hardship because of unforeseen illness. In terms of our other criteria, however, such plans must be judged unacceptable.

Although comprehensive insurance would remove the current incentive for patients to use inpatient rather than ambulatory care, it would not introduce any positive incentives for the efficient use of resources. Whatever cost consciousness is still existing today among patients, doctors, and administrators would be removed. There would be no incentive to limit the rising cost of hospital care, to use paramedical personnel more widely, or to produce physicians' services more efficiently. With all bills paid by the government, nothing would limit the rise in hospital wage rates and physicians' income. In such a situation, the government would be forced to introduce direct controls in an attempt to contain costs.

Such detailed controls, fee schedules, and limits on hospital charges might prevent rising costs for a while, but the experience of Canada, Britain, and Sweden suggests that health costs rise very rapidly even under government health programs with extensive direct controls. Such controls could not achieve, and might actually work against, an efficient use of health resources. They would certainly require a large number of arbitrary policy decisions and engender the hostility of the basic providers. Such arbitrary decisions pose more serious questions than may be generally recognized. What is a "reasonable" level of daily hospital cost? At what rate should hospitals improve facilities, add staff, or raise the level of amenities? How many beds should there be per thousand population? How much should different medical specialists earn? These are not technical questions that could be answered "objectively" if only enough research were done—they involve tastes and value judgments about the relative desirability of different goods and services.

Finally, even if expenditures were not to rise, the provision of comprehensive insurance would require a substantial tax increase: over $44 billion to replace current private expenditures on physician and hospital services, and an additional $34 billion if drugs and other personal health care were to be included.

If such a $78 billion increase in government spending were financed by increasing the tax rate of the current Social Security payroll tax, the rate would rise from its current level of 12 percent to more than 20 percent. If, instead, the $78 billion were financed by a general increase in the personal income tax, everyone's tax would have to rise by more than 50 percent of its current level.

Comprehensive insurance would shift the problem of the health-care sector to a conflict between cost inflation and controls. No matter where the balance between these was struck, there would be no natural incentive to efficiency, and there would be a large government expenditure to be paid for by much higher taxes.

The Major-Risk Approach

I favor a different approach to national health insurance. My proposal is extremely simple: Every family would receive a comprehensive major-risk insurance (MRI) policy with an annual "direct-expense limit"—i.e., a limit on out-of-pocket payments—that increases with family income. A $500 direct-expense limit means that the family is responsible for up to $500 of out-of-pocket medical expenses per year but pays no more than $500—no matter how large the total annul medical bill. Different relations between family income and the direct-expense limit are possible. For example, the expense limit might start at $400 per year for a family with income below $4,000, be equal to 10 percent of family income between $4,000 and $15,000, and be $1,500 for incomes above that level. The details of the schedule are unimportant at this point. The key feature is an expense limit that few families would normally exceed but that is low relative to family income.

Major-risk insurance is the most important type of health insurance for the government to provide. It concentrates government effort on those families for whom medical expenses would create financial hardship or preclude adequate care. Because relatively few families have such large expenditures in any year, MRI need not be a very costly program. In terms of our six criteria, these are the advantages of MRI:

1. *It would prevent deprivation of care.* If the maximum annual expenditure on health were limited to 10 percent or less of family income, no family would be deprived of care because of inability to pay. (If it is believed that certain types of preventive care and early diagnostic tests would not be undertaken as often as desirable, the MRI policy could be supplemented by specific coverage for these services at relatively little additional cost.)

2. *It would prevent financial hardship.* MRI would also prevent financial hardship by limiting a family's financial risk to 10 percent or less of annual income.

3. *It would reduce cost inflation.* An increase in insurance coverage generally exacerbates the inflation of hospital costs. However, the universal provision of MRI should reduce hospital-cost inflation by eliminating (or at least de-

creasing) the current use of shallow-coverage insurance. This would be particularly true if, in introducing national health insurance, the government eliminated the current tax subsidy for private health insurance. In any case, after MRI had removed the risk of major expense, families would then have little to gain from such insurance, for the cost of a policy would be high relative to the upper limit on expenses guaranteed by the MRI.

Of course, once a family had exceeded its direct-expense limit, MRI would be equivalent to comprehensive insurance, and the family would then have no incentive to limit its spending for medical care. To ensure that relatively few families do exceed their direct-expense limit, the MRI policy should make use of a coinsurance feature instead of a deductible. For example, the annual direct limit of $1,500 for families with incomes over $15,000 could be achieved by using a 50 percent coinsurance on the first $3,000 of medical bills. Fewer than one family in fifteen had medical expenses of more than $3,000 in 1976 (including, of course, the expenses now paid by insurance). Therefore, fewer than one famliy in fifteen would reach an expense limit that is based on $3,000 of spending. The coinsurance rates could be cut at lower income levels to keep the direct-expense limit to 10 percent of income, e.g., a 33 percent coinsurance rate at an income of $10,000. At some income level it would probably be desirable to cut the $3,000 base so that the coinsurance rate did not have to fall too drastically. It is encouraging in this regard that fewer than one family in five had 1976 expenses exceeding $1,500; a 30 percent coinsurance rate would produce a direct-expense limit of $450.

More discussion of these details is clearly out of place here. What I want to emphasize is the general principle: The combination of a coinsurance rate and an expenditure base can be selected in a way that varies with income to make almost all families significantly sensitive to the costs of additional health spending, while still limiting each family's maximum out-of-pocket expenditure to 10 percent of income or less.

Even for the small number of families who reach their limits, MRI would indirectly help to control expenditures. The basic cost per day in hospitals would not be determined by the willingness of those relatively few families to spend, but rather by the preferences of the far larger number of patients who would not be fully reimbursed. MRI could prevent excesses in physicians' fees and hospital durations of stay by requiring that the same care be given and the same fees be charged to these patients as to those who are paying for their care. Because most medical services would be financed with substantial direct payments, the standards of "customary charge" and "customary care" would become meaningful reference standards, as they currently are not. In short, MRI would introduce a cost-consciousness and a basis for cost comparison that could improve efficiency and contain medical-care inflation.

4. *It would avoid a large tax burden.* The cost to tax-payers of an MRI program would not be large relative to the benefits conferred. The exact amount would depend on the particular schedule of coinsurance and the overall impact of the program on utilization and unit costs. I would estimate that an MRI form of national health insurance that covered *all* personal health care would raise government spending by no more than $19 billion at 1976 levels. Limiting the scope of coverage or introducing a small deductible per spell of illness could reduce this cost more than proportionately.

5. *It would be administratively simple.* MRI would be relatively simple and inexpensive to administer. Because MRI would act to contain cost inflation and to increase efficiency, there would be no need for detailed controls or essentially arbitrary policy decisions. Planning efforts could be concentrated on those problems that cannot be solved by the natural forces of supply and demand.

6. *It would be generally acceptable.* An MRI scheme should be acceptable to physicians, hospitals, and the general public. It would have the virtue of providing full protection against serious financial hardship without the con-

trols or fee schedules that would accompany other forms of insurance. The current freedom of physicians and hospitals would be preserved. If MRI were administered by the same insurance companies that currently provide health insurance, the net effect would be a small increase in their total premium.

In conclusion, I want to reiterate that the problem of health care costs is not to *reduce* or to *limit* the growth of medical spending, but to achieve the *correct* rate of growth of that spending. In turn, this means that the form of national health insurance that the nation adopts should ensure that individual consumers play the central role in guiding the growth and form of their health services. I believe that MRI is the right way to protect families from the risk of financial hardship, while preserving individual freedom of choice and thereby making the future development of our health-care system responsive to the preferences of the people.

AMA PRESIDENT DISCUSSES
HEALTH-CARE COSTS [5]

Q: There has been a suggestion that all medical students have their training paid for completely by the government. They would be government employees, and after graduation they would be paid a salary determined by government and would be told where to practice medicine and under what conditions. What's wrong with this idea? Why should medicine be a free profession instead of a controlled public service?

A: That involves the very nature of a profession. One way I can answer that is to quote something Louis Brandeis wrote. [Brandeis was a Supreme Court Justice from 1916 to 1939.] "A profession is an occupation for which the neces-

[5] Excerpt from interview with Dr. Richard Palmer, president of American Medical Association (1976), by Sheila McGough, freelance writer. *National Observer.* p 12. Ap. 23, '77. Reprinted with permission of The National Observer, © Dow Jones & Company, Inc. 1977. All Rights Reserved.

sary preliminary training is intellectual in character, involving knowledge and to some extent learning as distinguished from a mere skill. It is an occupation that is pursued largely for others and not merely for oneself. It is an occupation in which the amount of financial remuneration is not the accepted measure of success."

Historically, the tremendous advances in medicine took place under the system of free professionals. This system does work. It has produced great benefits to many people. In fact, Senator Kennedy, who has been one of the severest critics of American medicine, made the statement that at its best, American medicine is the finest in the world. What Senator Kennedy fails to realize is that regulation by government is the very opposite of freedom. There must be a free interchange between patient and doctor. Otherwise we have lost the very heart and essence of the practice of medicine.

Q: We now have several examples of that kind of nationalized medicine, which Senator Kennedy and others seem to advocate. You are obviously against it, but do you have any evidence that it doesn't work well?

A: In the past several years I've been to the Peoples Republic of China. I've been to countries in South America, and Scandinavia, to Belgium, Germany, Switzerland, England, Bulgaria. And I just got back from the Soviet Union. In all these countries, with the possible exception of West Germany and Belgium, there is governmental control of medicine. The most disheartening example, I think, is Great Britain, where they have long queues of people waiting for simple operations. There's not enough money to run the system. The doctors are totally frustrated. They have said to me time and again in many of these countries: "For heaven's sake, can't your politicians see what has happened in our country? Can't they see that you have the best system for the practice of medicine and that you're doing the best job in the world? Can't they leave you alone?" [For information on the workings of national health insurance in England and in Sweden, see Section VII, below.]

Q: But specifically, from the standpoint of the patient, rather than the practitioner, what are some of the disadvantages of these national health systems?

A: There is virtually no freedom of choice. In Britain or Bulgaria or Russia, you're assigned a physician. And there's usually no way you can change that physician short of moving to another part of the country. This matter of choice is important. A sick human being is not like a broken machine. Any doctor can cite cases where a patient showed no improvement under one doctor's care, and then responded dramatically to exactly the same treatment from another, more compatible physician.

If the patient doesn't feel that he has a friend in the doctor sitting across the table from him, then we've lost the very essence of what a physician is supposed to do. And in countries like Great Britain it's rare that a physician will spend more than a very few minutes with a patient because of the overload of people waiting to see him. You see, whenever you have a tax-paid system, you have a hyped-up demand for care. Medicine, as I see it, is controlled by three factors: accessibility, cost, and quality of care. If you take any one of these three and alter it very much, you upset the delicately balanced troika. And the system will collapse.

For example, if you make the system too accessible through a tax-paid mechanism, then the doctors' offices are absolutely overrun with patients. Or, if you make the quality so high that the costs are unbearable—an example would be running exhaustive diagnostic tests every time a patient comes in with a head cold—then you limit the access so that people who really need medical treatment don't get it.

Q: In the United States today, how do you assess the accessibility, cost, and quality of health care? Are they in balance?

A: I think they are pretty well in balance right now. Older people are pretty well taken care of under Medicare. Treatment of the poor is provided through Medicaid. But some improvements could be made. Because of the differences in the Medicaid plans in each of the fifty states, there should be federalization of the Medicaid program so that the poor would have uniform benefits. For example, in Arizona there is no Medicaid program at all. Then we have the great in-between. It's our estimate that about 85 percent of those who are neither elderly nor poor have adequate health-care coverage through private insurance. [See "Why Rural Doctors Are Missing," above, in Section IV, for another view of this question.]

Looking at these facts, we have endorsed a bill introduced by Congressman [T.L. Carter] of Kentucky and Senator [Clifford] Hansen of Wyoming. It would provide basic comprehensive health care, including care for catastrophic illness or injury to all patients. It would be based upon the existing private insurance mechanisms. It would not build a new bureaucracy. It would limit government control to the absolute minimum.

There would be free choice of physician. There would be a pluralistic delivery system, including solo practitioners, group practices, and health maintenance organizations. The employer would be mandated to offer the insurance to his employees. They would share the expenses, with the employer paying the larger portion, about 65 percent. Less federal money would be needed to implement this plan than for any other now in the hopper.

Q: What about people who are unemployed?

A: Their insurance would be paid by the federal government out of general funds. Part of the plan is to have the federal government take over the Medicaid program. Someone who lost his job would have his health insurance carried for a month or so by his previous employer, and then he would either be enrolled in his new employer's insurance plan or, if he remained unemployed, become eligible for Medicaid benefits.

Q: Those who support a federal health-insurance system, like the one sponsored by Senator Kennedy, say that one big advantage of having the government pay for all health care is that the government would then be able to impose strict cost controls, and that would save the medical consumer a lot of money. What's your response to that?

A: With the Carter-Hansen bill we would have built in a form of quality control—peer review, ultilization review—within the profession. You have to remember, too, in the Kennedy proposal we would really be getting a national health service instead of just national health insurance. It would be very much like the British plan. All the fees would be paid out of taxes, and this would necessitate a huge tax increase.

Q: Do you think many people have an unrealistic expectation of what they can get from their doctor or hospital or other medical care provider?

A: Perhaps so. They have a right to expect a great deal from medicine, and more knowledge is continually being added. But good health still requires prudence and self-discipline on the part of the patient and cooperation with his doctor and other health professionals. I want to emphasize that American medicine as it is practiced today is the finest in the world, and it's being done almost entirely in the private sector.

VI. HEALTH MAINTENANCE ORGANIZATIONS

EDITOR'S INTRODUCTION

One of the Nixon Administration's contributions to the containment of medical care costs was a 1973 law that promoted the development of health maintenance organizations (HMOs). HMOs—actually corporations consisting of a group of doctors working together—control costs by offering to provide medical care to individuals and families at a set annual fee. If a member of an HMO requires expensive surgery, it costs the HMO money. Thus, it's in the HMO's interest to prevent major illnesses by maintaining the health of its members.

The best-known and most successful HMO is the Kaiser-Permanente Health Plan, described in this section's first article taken from *Dun's Review*. The second piece, "Containing the Cost of Employee Health Plans," reprinted from *Business Week*, demonstrates the attraction of these plans for businesses that underwrite the medical care of their employees. Each year, General Motors spends more on medical care than it does on steel. The HMO concept promises to help large companies such as General Motors to hold down their share of employees' medical bills.

But HMOs have drawbacks, too. County medical societies tend to view them as competitors to local doctors paid in the traditional fee-for-service manner and thus tend to resist them. The American Medical Association has pressured more than a dozen state legislatures into outlawing such plans even while being prosecuted under antitrust laws for trying to kill prepaid plans in other states. Furthermore, HMOs are not always popular with their members, as this section's final excerpt, "Less May Be Enough," from *National Review*, makes clear.

KAISER AND THE "DESERT DOCTORS":
A WAY TO CUT MEDICAL BILLS [1]

When seven construction companies dispatched five thousand men to build the Grand Coulee Dam in the remote northeastern corner of Washington State in 1938, they faced innumerable problems of supporting the crew. Not the least was the task of providing medical care. The solution to the dilemma, largely the work of Henry J. Kaiser, was an imaginative arrangement that has grown into one of the country's most successful health-care programs. And as the nation today examines the staggering costs of medical care, the plan born thirty-nine years ago on the banks of the Columbia River has become increasingly attractive.

On-the-Job MDs

Kaiser, the principal contractor on the project, persuaded his partners to take over, refurbish and air condition a seventy-five-bed hospital near the dam site; they also hired the "desert doctors," a team headed by Los Angeles physician Sidney Garfield, who a few years earlier had set up a hospital on skids and followed construction workers as they built an aqueduct from the Colorado River to Los Angeles. Kaiser and the other contractors paid the doctors a lump sum in advance, and the doctors agreed to treat the workers for on-the-job accidents. The unions and the workers themselves paid an additional advance fee to cover other accidents and illnesses: seven cents a day for each worker, seven cents for his wife and twenty-five cents a week for children.

That was the beginning of the Kaiser-Permanente Medical program (Permanente is the name of a creek in the Santa Cruz Mountains that caught the fancy of Kaiser's first wife.) During World War II, the plan was extended to Kaiser shipyards and the Kaiser steel mill on the West Coast,

[1] Article by Lee Smith, senior editor. *Dun's Review.* 109:23+. My. '77. Reprinted with the special permission of *Dun's Review*, May 1977. Copyright, 1977, Dun & Bradstreet Publications Corporation.

and after the war it was opened up to people other than Kaiser employees. Today, it has 3.1 million subscribers in California, Oregon, Washington, Hawaii, Colorado and Ohio. Among its largest clients are government agencies, labor unions and such corporations as Ford, General Motors and Ohio Bell Telephone. Less than 2 percent of its members are Kaiser employees, and the Kaiser Foundation Health Plan, Inc., and Kaiser Foundation Hospitals, which administer the program, are entities separate from Kaiser Industries.

Kaiser Permanente differs from organizations such as Blue Cross and Blue Shield; it is not an insurer that reimburses others for services, but an actual provider of health care. Kaiser-Permanente owns and operates 26 community hospitals with 5,711 beds, and also 66 outpatient clinics. It employs 3,000 full-time physicians and 25,000 nurses, technicians, administrators and other aides. The doctors agree to work for a predetermined salary, but if they provide the care at less than budget, they get a share of the surplus. And if they go over their budget, they have to make up the difference.

A subscriber pays in advance a set fee that varies somewhat according to the section of the country and whether or not the member is single or has a family. A single subscriber in the San Francisco area pays $23.95 a month, and this entitles him or her to a complete range of medical care, from an unlimited number of trips to the outpatient clinic to 365 days a year in a hospital for everything from a routine checkup to intensive cancer care and open-heart surgery. A subscriber with a spouse pays $47.70 and with children as well, $67.62. The plan will also reimburse other doctors and hospitals if the member gets sick while traveling. In most regions, there are extra charges for dental care and eyeglasses; psychiatric consultation is included in the plan but not psychiatric hospitalization; there is a $60 charge for routine maternity care, and there is a fee for house calls: $3.50 if the doctor comes in the morning: $5 in the afternoon.

The Drawbacks

The plan has its drawbacks. For one thing, a patient has little choice as to doctor or hospital. Also, it seems best suited for metropolitan areas, where there are enough subscribers to justify hospitals with a full range of services, and a staff with a broad array of specialties. Still, for four decades the plan has demonstrated that good medical care can be provided for a cost that can be kept under control. A single subscriber to the Kaiser-Permanente plan in San Francisco, for example, pays about 50 percent less than a subscriber to the Blue Cross hospital and major medical plan and yet receives more service. Blue Cross covers only 80 percent of hospital costs and doctors' fees and pays nothing at all for such incidentals as routine physical checkups.

Last year [1976], the plan collected $907 million, most of it in advance, from its subscribers and paid out $866 million for services. That left it with a net income of $41 million to be invested in new buildings and equipment. As Edgar F. Kaiser, chairman of both Kaiser Industries and the Kaiser health organizations, has expressed it: "When history records my father's accomplishments, the emphasis will be on the medical care program."

CONTAINING THE COST OF EMPLOYEE HEALTH PLANS—WITH HEALTH MAINTENANCE ORGANIZATIONS [2]

Bynum E. Tudor, director of employee benefits for R.J. Reynolds Industries Inc. in Winston-Salem, North Carolina, used to worry a lot about the rising cost of the company's health insurance program—20 percent higher each year, with no end in sight. "We had no control over our health insurance system whatsoever," Tudor says.

Today Tudor feels a great deal better. Reynolds has gone into the health-care business on its own, competing

[2] Article in *Business Week*. p 74-6. My. 30, '77. Reprinted from the May 30, 1977 issue of *Business Week* by special permission. © 1977 by McGraw-Hill, Inc.

successfully with its long-time health insurance contractor, Blue Cross. Some 10,000 employees and their family members have chosen the company's health-care program over their former insurer and 13,000 are on a waiting list. Moreover, after less than a year, RJR reports that the program costs less per employee than Blue Cross premiums for comparable coverage.

The program that erased the furrows from Tudor's brow is the Winston-Salem Health Care Plan Inc., one of some 180 health maintenance organizations (HMOs) that provide 7 million subscribers with a comprehensive range of health services for flat monthly fees. Family members get treatment for everything from junior's sniffles to dad's coronary arrest in or out of a hospital. Their monthly fee covers all charges. Long a theoretical alternative to conventional health insurance (and, in a few areas, a sturdily functioning one), HMOs have suddenly become the country's hottest concept in health care, thanks largely to business interest. And while RJR may be the only corporation to run an HMO exclusively for its employees, HMOs are being talked up in board rooms from coast to coast—most recently, and fervently, in Detroit, where Ford Motor Company has backed a feasibility study by experts from the big brother of all HMOs, the 3.1-million-member nonprofit Kaiser Foundation Health Plan.

A Lengthening List

Companies that already offer the HMO option to their employees include the Big Three auto makers, American Telephone & Telegraph, General Mills, Dow Chemical, Bechtel, Alcoa, Sherwin-Williams, Sears Roebuck, Xerox, IBM, Sun Company, Bell & Howell, and a lengthening list of others. US Steel, J. C. Penney, and American Can have joined the list just this year [1977]. PepsiCo plans to offer the option within the next few months.

Says Lawrence P. Carrington, manager of planning and development at AT&T: "HMOs are doing the job for us that we wanted done." AT&T began offering the HMO option back in 1972. The 8 percent of its 75,000 employees who chose it, says Carrington, "are probably getting better health care than the ones who didn't, at less expense to AT&T both in terms of benefit costs and in sick time lost."

Carrington's remarks are typical. Companies that offer HMO membership report almost universally that the system controls costs by drastically cutting the number and length of hospital stays: first, because its emphasis on preventive care produces fewer seriously sick patients and, second, because the flat-fee formula discourages doctors from hospitalizing patients unnecessarily or keeping them hospitalized longer than necessary. Some HMO groups log half the hospital days of comparable insured groups. Employers also like the fact that prepaid plans enable them to budget health-care costs to the penny. And—the clincher for many companies—as the traditional health insurance providers raise their rates by as much as 50 percent a year, the cost advantages they formerly enjoyed over most HMOs are narrowing or disappearing.

Favorable Trend

The situation varies plan by plan. Health Care Louisville Inc. in Kentucky charges $72.90 a month for family coverage, higher than the Blues' rate of $62.95, while the Rutgers Community Health Plan in New Brunswick, New Jersey, charges $60.69, $12 below the Blues' rate. But the long haul seems to favor the HMOs, whose costs are rising more slowly than those of the insurers. Kaiser's John J. Boardman Jr. believes that, on average, "the cost lines have crossed during the past two years." In northern California, Kaiser undercuts the Blues by 20 percent or more.

As the country's biggest and best-known HMO, Kaiser has received so many industry requests for advice that it recently created a management consultant firm, Kaiser-Permanente Advisory Services, with Boardman as director. Ford contracted with the group, says Jack K. Shelton, manager of Ford's employee-insurance department, because company health-care costs were doubling every five years, to the current annual total of $460 million, and a national study had shown that HMO costs averaged significantly below those of conventional Blue Cross and Blue Shield plans. The 5 percent of Ford's own employees who belong to HMOs (including one in Detroit) cost the company less than those served by the Blues, says Shelton. If Ford gets the go-ahead, he says, the auto maker will back the creation of a second Detroit-area HMO.

Mandatory Alternative

Within the next few years, the company that does not offer its employees the opportunity to join an HMO will probably be the exception rather than the rule. Under the "dual option" provision of the 1973 HMO law, every company with twenty-five or more employees must offer HMO membership as an alternative to its current employee health insurance plan if a federally qualified HMO exists in the vicinity. Congress set this requirement to help foster the growth of HMOs, protecting employers from being penalized for their foster-parent role by asking them to pay only the sum they normally paid for health insurance if the HMO membership fee ran higher. The employee himself would pay the difference.

But HMOs, potentially a $5 billion industry, failed to grow beyond their established 5 percent of the market because the 1973 law contained a Catch-22 provision. It demanded that federally certified HMOs provide so many services—ophthalmology, mental health care, dentistry for children—that few HMOs could qualify. Any that tried would wind up being far too expensive to compete with conventional insurance.

Last June [1976] Congress amended the law, reducing HMO service qualifications to manageable proportions and easing enrollment requirements that might have stuck HMOs with an outsize load of elderly and infirm members. Companies did not even wait for President Ford to sign the bill last fall. The National Association of Employers on Health Maintenance Organizations (NAEHMO) held its founding meeting in Minneapolis in July, and the business campaign to promote HMOs was under way.

Today the Health, Education & Welfare Department has certified only 30 of the nation's 180 HMOs, but additional ones are seeking certification and employers, consumer groups, and even traditional health insurers are announcing plans for new groups. Less than a year after its formation, the NAEHMO has 117 member companies interested in creating or working with HMOs.

"Cost Containment"

The companies join, says Ruth H. Stack, executive director, both because of the dual option requirement and out of "a very real concern about health costs, period." Under conventional health insurance, NAEHMO member companies experienced an average annual 23 percent increase in their health-care packages during the past two years.

Traditional insurers, who can spot a trend as well as anyone else, have also boarded the bandwagon. The Health Insurance Association of America reports that 22 insurance companies are involved in 50 HMOs in 25 states, and the Blues sponsor, administer, market, or have some other link with 107 HMOs. Insurers say they see no conflict between their promotion of traditional plans and their promotion of HMOs. In Rochester, New York, the Blues simultaneously underwrite and manage two HMOs and sell standard health insurance. "We provide the community's mechanisms for paying health care, leaving the choice to the public," says Donald Robertson, president of the Rochester Blue Shield.

Both HMOs are prospering with a combined membership of 110,000 in a field where 30,000 members are usually considered the breakeven point. A third Rochester HMO fell by the wayside.

This high breakeven point represents the HMOs' major obstacle and also explains their need for well-heeled sponsors. Without solid financial backing, the plans face the circular dilemma of attracting members fast enough to pay the high startup costs of acquiring the staff and equipment that will attract members. As a result, only a few HMOs have done more than squeak by. Some 90 percent of all HMO members belong to only twenty plans, and those twenty tend to have substantial patrons. Typically, the United Auto Workers founded Detroit's 76,000-member Metro Health Plan and ran it for five years before turning it over to the Blues. The Kaiser plan alone accounts for almost half of HMO membership, 2,617,000 in California and 483,000 in four other states.

The Kaiser Foundation, the HMO everyone knows, was founded in 1933 by industrialist Henry J. Kaiser, originally to provide his employees with medical facilities at construction sites that lacked them. The plans took their characteristic form, says Dr. Sidney Garfield, one of the planners, because the men working on their design rapidly discovered that "much of the high cost of medical care was due to waste resulting from poorly planned facilities, insufficient coordination between physicians and the institution in which they worked, and insufficient coordination between physician and physician. The simple solution was to bring the physicians into coordinated group practice, operating a medical center geared to serve them efficiently."

Salaried Doctors

Kaiser expanded during World War II, opened its rolls to outsiders in 1945, and the rest is history. The foundation adds several new centers each year, paid $80.5 million for capital expenditures last year [1976], and employs 3,137 salaried doctors—who, like most HMO doctors, earn somewhat less than many of their peers in private practice, but follow their calling undistracted by paper work and call their lives their own after office hours.

What is civilized living for doctors, however, is a marketing problem for most HMOs. Many potential members fear that they will encounter an unfamiliar doctor in an emergency. HMOs have tried to accommodate this reaction by introducing some flexibility into scheduling. They also stress that private-practice doctors, too, sometimes refer their patients to substitutes.

Realistically, however, the private-practice doctor loses money with every substitution and the HMO doctor usually does not. Against this must be balanced the fact that the private-practice doctor usually makes money with every visit and procedure, necessary or unnecessary, and the HMO doctor does not.

Since HMOs come in a variety of forms, some doctors have it both ways. As participants in foundation HMOs, doctors may serve some patients on a prepaid basis—usually drawing a lesser "fee" for each visit from the foundation and sharing whatever gains or losses remain at yearend with their colleagues—and treat other patients on a conventional fee-for-service basis.

The typical HMO, however, resembles any other suite of offices occupied by a large group of physicians practicing different specialties. Often it includes laboratories. Unlike the Kaiser plan, which runs its own hospitals, it refers members to hospitals and other special facilities under contract to the HMO. Doctors have hospital staff privileges, just as they would in private practice.

A Plan Evolves

RJR Industries, which certainly never expected to find itself running an HMO, embarked on the path to the Winston-Salem Health Care Plan five years ago when it decided to investigate the causes of rising health insurance costs. Its task force made one discovery after another. Because of the shortage of doctors in the area, some 45 percent of the company's 14,000 employees simply reported to hospital emergency rooms for medical care, says RJR's Tudor. "It cost something like $45 for those people just to walk through the door," he adds. Moreover, some employees remained hospitalized for suspiciously long periods. Tudor recalls one seven-week stay for a condition that normally requires ten days' hospitalization.

Turning to the search for solutions, officials visited some HMOs and, says Tudor, "after that, it wasn't a question of whether or not this was our alternative, but how to start one." The Winston-Salem Health Care Plan opened last summer [1976] with much hoopla and 6,000 members, all it could accommodate immediately, of the 23,000 employees and dependents who asked to join. It is still interviewing doctors—one thousand have applied at "highly competitive salaries," says Tudor—and expects to have facilities for 19,000 members by yearend. The company counts on recouping its $2 million in startup costs within two years. Meanwhile, Tudor says, "The facility is giving our people high-quality medical care for about half the price of Blue Cross." Equally important, he says, "The plan permits us some control over the quality of what we pay for."

In Minneapolis, officials of General Mills Inc. express similar enthusiasm. The company gave its employees the HMO option four years ago, has 57 percent of its work force signed up today, and reports happily that the employees who belong to HMOs average half the hospital days of the other employees.

Other Appproaches

But not all company reports are upbeat. The three auto makers in Detroit note that the percentage of their workers enrolled in the Detroit Metro Health Plan has declined as workers moved to the suburbs. And in Akron, Goodyear Tire & Rubber Company feels that active involvement in local health-delivery systems may do more to keep down costs than sponsorship of HMOs in areas where health-care capacity exceeds demand.

Not even Tudor believes that HMOs are likely to replace all the employer health insurance, which covers 140 million workers and their dependents. But most observers would agree with him that they will inevitably play a large role in companies' efforts to control employee health-care costs because of their built-in bias toward economy.

"The biggest asset a hospital or doctor has is sick people," says Tudor. "The biggest asset an HMO has is healthy people. HMOs reap economic rewards for keeping people well. That's why they work for business."

LESS MAY BE ENOUGH [3]

With the cost of health care consistently going up, many people have turned to medical insurance programs like Blue Cross–Blue Shield to help cope with the bills, but these programs are by no means the only plans available. A comparatively new method of paying for and guaranteeing medical care has been receiving much attention: the prepaid group plan, in which those affiliated with the plan pay a flat fee in advance and are guaranteed treatment. On the face of it, it isn't obvious why this method should be able to reduce expenses. There might be some savings and convenience in grouping several specialists under one roof, so that they can share facilities, but this can be (and often is) combined with fees that vary according to use. Yet it seems the prepaid plan does work. In 1967 the National Advisory Commission on Health Manpower examined the Kaiser Plan, the largest prepaid plan, and found the cost of the average member's medical care was "20 to 30 percent less than it would be if he obtained it outside."

Prepaid plans like the Kaiser Plan not only cost less, they also deliver less—but less may be enough. A study of the Federal Employees Health Benefits Program for 1966 found that 98 of every 1,000 Blue Cross–Blue Shield patients were hospitalized, compared to 46 of every 1,000 prepaid-group members. Blue Cross–Blue Shield patients spent 876 days in the hospital, compared to 408 for the group members. There were 73 operations per 1,000 Blue Shield subscribers, 31 per 1,000 among group-practice patients.

This helps solve the mystery of why prepaid health-care plans keep people equally healthy for less money. First of

[3] Excerpt from "The High Cost of Health," by Alan Reynolds, freelance writer. *National Review*. 25:782–3. Jl 20, '73. Reprinted by permission of *National Review*, 150 E. 35th St., New York, NY 10016

all, prepaid plans have a much lower ratio of surgeons to patients than does the nation as a whole (1 surgeon for 10,000 to 17,000, versus 1 for every 7,554 nationally), and, since patients pay a flat rate regardless of treatment, unnecessary surgery or hospitalization means more work for the surgeon or hospital, which doesn't bring in any extra income. Medicare and Blue Cross-Blue Shield, on the other hand, encourage hospitalization even for routine tests, and the income of fee-for-service surgeons is directly related to the number of operations they perform. The variation in surgical treatment between conventional and prepaid plans, and among regions, prompted the pseudonymous surgeon who wrote *How To Avoid Unnecessary Surgery* to estimate that one operation in five is unnecessary. Dr. John Knowles, President of the Rockefeller Foundation, was censured for saying what the statistics tell us must be true: "Three to four doctors out of ten are either doing unnecessary surgery or are overcharging." Moreover, prepaid plans do not usually charge higher income patients more. This is why the AMA has pressured seventeen states into outlawing such plans, and has been prosecuted under antitrust laws for trying to kill prepaid plans in other states.

Price discrimination, padded lab bills, and unnecessary surgery are not inherent features of fee-for-service medical care. They are a direct result of monopoly and enforced secrecy—particularly the suppression of price information and advertising. Prepaid plans don't really get to the root of this problem, nor of such problems as the oversupply of surgeons. For example, if there were more prepaid plans, the ratio of surgeons to the population *outside* those plans would become even higher, because the prepaid plans employ fewer surgeons per covered population, leaving more surgeons per capita outside the groups.

Prepaid group practice has other problems of its own. A family of three under the Kaiser Plan now pays up to $600 a year regardless of use—quite a lot more than many families (including my own) spend on medical expenses and insurance. And Kaiser facilities are indeed large, but they

are also few and far between. Improving access by building
more facilities, particularly in rural areas, might eliminate
the economies of a large, factory-like operation. Kaiser patients complain about the difficulty in getting appointments, and about having to wait for doctors they don't
know. When they do get to see their doctor, the visit is a
short one, since the doctors are scheduled to see a patient
every fifteen minutes—barely enough time to prescribe two
aspirin and plenty of rest.

VII. MODELS FROM ABROAD

EDITOR'S INTRODUCTION

No volume on medical care would be complete without a look at the way foreign countries organize their systems of health care. The United States can learn much from the experience of other nations. In fact, Secretary Joseph A. Califano of the United States Department of Health, Education, and Welfare has already made at least one trip to Canada to study that nation's medical care program. In 1958 Canada adopted a national hospital-insurance program to cover all Canadians. Ten years later it adopted a national insurance plan to cover doctors' services.

This section focuses on two different systems. The first selection, by Joseph G. Simanis, economist in the Social Security Administration, examines the British National Health Service. The NHS is not, strictly speaking, an insurance plan. It is a highly centralized system with doctors, dentists, and other professionals on its payroll. These public servants provide their services to patients at no direct charge to the patient.

The second selection, taken from *JAMA*, the Journal of the American Medical Association, and written by Dr. Joseph L. Andrews Jr., explores medical care in Sweden, where the system is financed largely by a national insurance plan. When a Swede goes to a hospital, the government picks up the bill. But the government and the patient share the cost of doctors' fees and drugs. The system is extremely costly in taxes and the Swedish people are grumbling about both this and the impersonality of the care.

Interesting as these two systems are, it seems very unlikely that either one will ever be transplanted to the United States. Fee-for-service medicine, dominated by health professionals, is the system that Americans know best and trust the most. Few experts on medical care in America foresee any national health insurance plan changing that. But most do foresee change in other areas—to control costs and to make medical care accessible to everyone in the nation.

THE BRITISH NATIONAL HEALTH SERVICE [1]

When it was introduced in 1948, the National Health Service of the United Kingdom, which provided health care to the whole population, represented a breakthrough. Only a few other countries had universal coverage. New Zealand began phasing in its universal system in 1939; the Soviet Union also provided health care to its whole population. The United Kingdom, nonetheless, was the first major industrialized Western country to introduce a health system accessible to all its people. The National Health Service was not the country's first government program—a national health insurance system had been launched in 1912 —but by 1948 it still covered only 40 percent of the population.

Most West European countries and Japan also had national health programs; but for the most part they were insurance schemes covering only a portion of the population, similar to the one which the United Kingdom had just abandoned. As late as 1955, for instance, the French and Belgian systems covered only 48 and 53 percent of the population, respectively. Subsequently, however, coverage was extended in those countries and is now virtually universal in all of them. Australia and Canada have also moved toward universal coverage.

In West Europe, the Netherlands is an exception to this pattern of nearly universal coverage for medical care, because only 76 percent of the population has access to a full range of health services that are essentially free under the general health-care program. The portion of the population

[1] From article by Joseph G. Simanis, economist, Office of Research and Statistics, U.S. Social Security Administration. *Current History.* 73:27–9+. Jl./Ag. '77. Copyright © 1977 by Current History, Inc. Reprinted by permission.

excluded, however, is essentially made up of higher income groups who are expected to contract for private health insurance to cover the expenses of their health care. Even this excluded portion of the population has been covered for catastrophic types of illness in a special, universal program inaugurated in 1967.

The United States is also an exception in the prevailing pattern of universal coverage in the developed world. Its national health program now covers only the aged and certain categories of the disabled, roughly about 10 percent of the population.

The British Experience

A national health service is a form of health-care delivery that provides comprehensive services that are either free at the point of delivery or involve a minimum of cost sharing by the patient. Funds are generally provided by the government out of general tax revenue. Widespread public ownership of medical facilities is usually, but not always, a feature of the system. Doctors in most cases are employed by the government, but here again there are exceptions.

General practitioners in the United Kingdom, for instance, are self-employed professionals paid on a modified capitation basis. For ambulatory care, New Zealand's national health service depends primarily on private doctors, who receive a flat payment from the government for each consultation and bill the patient for the remainder of their fee. In New Zealand (and in France) copayments required of a patient may be substantial, but the program is designed so that serious and costly illnesses do not place a heavy burden on the patient.

Early proponents of Britain's National Health Service predicted that costs would decline after the inception of the program, because improved access to health care would result in improved health, lower morbidity, and a subsequent decrease in the demand for health service. Although utilization never dropped, costs rose only modestly in the early years of the program and, as a share of rising GNP (gross national product), costs actually declined from 4.2 percent in 1950 to 3.6 percent in 1954. They remained relatively stable for a few years and then began to rise again, reaching 4.1 percent of GNP in 1960. . . .

In 1973, . . . the share of GNP devoted to health by the United Kingdom had risen to 5.3 percent, in other countries the share had risen to even higher percentages. The United States spent 7.7 percent of its GNP for health care, Sweden, 7.0 percent, and the Netherlands, 7.3 percent. . . .

Controls and Rationing

Among the specific areas of health-care delivery in which the National Health Service seems to have succeeded in keeping costs down is the pharmaceutical field. In this connection, after conducting a study of several countries, R. K. Schicke concluded that Great Britain has relatively low unit-costs and utilization levels for pharmaceuticals and, as a consequence, has relatively low overall per capita expenditures. Abel-Smith [Brian Abel-Smith, professor of social administration, University of London, at London School of Economics, author of many studies on health costs and their trends] attributes the relatively low costs to the central negotiation of prices with manufacturing suppliers, conducted against a background of possible legislative sanctions. In the National Health Service, a review system that monitors the prescribing practices of individual doctors also probably plays a role. If a family doctor's prescribing cost exceeds the average for other doctors in his area by 25 percent, he may be asked to explain his procedures. Although few doctors are ever disciplined as a result, the system reminds doctors of the need for economy.

Traditionally, the pharmaceuticals have represented a little over 8 percent of the National Health Service expenditures. For purposes of comparison, in 1973 in France expenditures on pharmaceuticals represented 23 percent of total personal health expenditures.

The relatively low income of personnel engaged in health services in the British system also provides economies. A recent study shows that of the nine countries in the Common Market, doctors' salaries are lowest in Great Britain. In 1973, general practitioners there earned only about one third of the income received by their counterparts in the Netherlands and Germany (and in the United States).

British nurses are also paid relatively low salaries, receiving less than the national average wage in manufacturing; ancillary workers in the hospitals are among the poorest paid in the country. It is possible, however, that Britain will follow the pattern established in other industrialized countries and that, in time, hospital workers will upgrade their relatively poor status in earnings and become relatively well paid.

The third area in which the National Health System seems to have established low expenditure levels is in capital investments. For the most part, there has been little building of hospitals in Britain over the past few decades. As a result, physical plant is antiquated. There was some improvement in the 1960s, but in 1973 the government cut back expenditures extensively, in line with other economies. Projections for capital expenditures through the 1970s indicate reduced activity in the field of hospital construction.

The low level of hospital construction has contributed to the shortage of hospital beds in Britain. As a result, a patient may wait a long time for elective surgery. Although waiting lists supposedly do not apply to urgent cases and are only in effect for discretionary surgery, there are apparently exceptions. Thus Michael H. Cooper notes that, for a certain type of brain surgery, children in the Liverpool-Warrington area have encountered a two- or three-year waiting period. During this period, their condition can deteriorate appreciably.

The shortage of funds also affects technological development. As of 1973, for instance, only a fraction of those patients who could benefit from lifesaving renal dialysis were provided with this service. Cooper questions whether optional allocation of resources in this regard has been achieved.

In general, a rather stringent rationing of resources is apparently involved in the more or less successful curbing of costs, particularly with respect to capital expenditures. Some apologists for the National Health Service maintain that, in establishing priorities and in negotiating with doctors, hospital workers and drug manufacturers, a single central authority provides a greater opportunity to counter inflationary demands.

The basic alternative to the national health service approach in health care is national health insurance. The insurance approach is perhaps best exemplified in West Germany, pioneer of all national health programs, which traces its system to 1883. About 90 percent of the population in the Federal Republic is covered, usually all except the higher income groups, who have chosen private coverage instead. The system is funded primarily by joint employer-employee payroll contributions. Most doctors are in private practice and, although most hospital accommodations are in public institutions, the private sector also plays a major role in the country's hospital care. Small copayments are required for drug prescriptions, for some forms of dental work, and for orthopedics. Doctors are generally paid according to a binding fee schedule, based on government guidelines and negotiated for specifics between representatives of the doctors on the one hand and the health insurance organizations on the other.

According to this method, every calendar quarter each Sickness Insurance Fund pays a lump sum to the local doctors' association for the provision of needed health care to insured members and dependents. The overall amount is negotiated between the fund and the association. At the end of the quarter, the association divides the lump sum among the doctors according to the services rendered. If the doctors generate more services than had been estimated, they receive a lower reimbursement per service. It is assumed that this method deters an individual doctor from generating more services than necessary, or more costly services than necessary, since he would then be increasing his income at the expense of his colleagues. The doctors' associations also monitor payments to make sure that the volume of claims and the form of treatment meet established norms. . . .

In most advanced countries today, the literature related to health care often speaks of a crisis in rising costs, reflecting a universal concern with this problem. The United Kingdom is no exception. Nonetheless, the British system has encountered relatively less of an increase than other countries. . . .

On balance, researchers who have treated the subject in depth maintain that British health care measures up adequately in comparison with other countries, where the reality also departs from the ideal. For instance, although it is recognized that the United Kingdom's capitation approach encourages primary doctors to refer their patients, sometimes unnecessarily, to specialists, critics of the fee-for-service approach argue that such a system encourages unnecessary treatments, including dangerous and costly surgery.

In response to the suggestion sometimes encountered that the United Kingdom does not spend enough on health care to maintain high standards, writers like Abel-Smith cite the available data on crude health indicators. In fact, Abel-Smith concludes that the level of health expenditures in advanced countries has little relation to the health status of the population, at least as measured by crude health indicators. Cooper notes that much of the progress in health care must be credited to environmental and economic factors rather than to providers of health services. Dr. Kerr White [educator, physician, editor, and writer] suggests that only about 20 percent of medical procedures in any country are truly useful; the others, at best, serve a placebo function.

The British National Health Service pioneered in providing universal, high-quality health care with a comprehensive range of benefits dispensed free at the point of delivery. While most other industrialized countries now also have universal coverage under their health-care systems, only a few provide a full range of services free or at nominal charge.

The British system seems to have been relatively successful in containing rising costs of health-care delivery and, on balance, in maintaining standards. Much of this success, however, seems to be due to the stringent rationing of resources by a central government authority, to the detriment of some suppliers and some patients. Rationing in some form is a necessary part of all health systems. Yet there are so many variations in health-care programs and approaches that it is reasonable to presume the possibility of better solutions. The situation warrants more research in order to determine and evaluate a wide range of alternative approaches to the provision of health care.

MEDICAL CARE IN SWEDEN [2]

Sweden is often cited as having one of the best medical care systems in the world. Admirers of the system point to the planning and organization that make high-quality health care available to all Swedish citizens, regardless of cost, and have made Sweden one of the healthiest nations of the world. When assessed by many indices of health, such as its infant-survival rate—the highest in the world, or its longevity rate—the second highest in the world, Sweden is ahead of many other nations, including the United States, which ranks eighteenth in the infant-survival rates and twenty-second in life expectancy.

On the other hand, critics have claimed that the Swedish national medical system provides care that is impersonal and second rate. They see increasing socialization as weakening the system further by increasing patient demands,

[2] Article by Dr. Joseph L. Andrews Jr. *JAMA* (Journal of the American Medical Association). 223:1369–75. Mr. 19, '73. Copyright 1973, American Medical Association. Reprinted by permission.

costs, and thus taxes while lessening personal incentive, thereby increasing existing shortages of doctors, nurses, and medical facilities.

How does the Swedish health-care system really work? How effective is it? How happy are patients and doctors? What changes have taken place recently and what will change in the future? Accurate answers to these questions are crucial before any comparisons can be made between Swedish and American medicine and before we can determine what features of the Swedish health-care system America should adopt and which we should avoid.

I spent two months in Gothenburg (Göteborg), Sweden's second largest city, visiting medical facilities and talking to medical personnel and patients at all levels. What I found is based on observations, conversations, and material written by Swedes most involved in health care.

Historical Background

Sweden is slightly larger than California in area and provides land for more than eight million Swedes. Resources of iron ore, forests, and water power combined with technologic skill have created a prosperous mixed economy in the mid-twentieth century and have helped to erase the poverty of the early 1900s. The government owns the railroads, iron mines, and television stations, but most factories and retail stores are privately owned. Government medicine predominates but private practice still exists.

Thus, these characteristics of Sweden—a homogeneous people, a long tradition of culture and government, more than 150 years of peace, a prosperous mixed industrial economy, and over forty years of socialist political dominance—form the important background for understanding the country's unique developments in social welfare and medical care.

Development of Medical Care: Social Insurance. As Sweden emerged from a poor agricultural economy to a more prosperous industrial economy in the earlier parts of the twentieth century, many workers, retaining memories of poverty in their youth, supported the Social-Democrat party whose main goal during its forty years of power has been to enact public measures that would protect all citizens against threats of insecurity and illness. Sweden's National Social Insurance covers every aspect of life from maternity benefits to old-age pensions at age sixty-seven. The emphasis on social welfare has changed from the turn-of-the-century concept of "helping people to help themselves" to the gradual assumption by the public sector of the responsibility for organizing and to a large extent financing a system that offers insurance against sickness, disability, and old age.

Before 1955, health insurance was voluntary. In 1955 the Swedish National Health Insurance created national compulsory tax-financed health insurance and in 1963, health insurance was combined with various pensions into the National Social Insurance Act.

Now the health insurance section of the National Social Insurance provides for all Swedes:

1. *Hospital Care.* Total coverage for unlimited periods for care at government hospitals including room charges, the attendance of staff doctors, surgery, laboratory and X-ray film charges (includes medical fees as well), and all drugs. (Almost all hospitals are financed and run by the county councils.)

2. *Sickness Benefits.* For wage earners, proportional to their salary levels.

3. *Ambulatory Care.* Partial reimbursement of doctors' fees, drugs, and the patient's traveling expenses. In January 1970, the "Seven Crown Reform," a new payment scheme for the ambulatory care provided by the county councils, was introduced. In essence, the patient now pays the first seven crowns (about $1.40) himself for each outpatient visit, while the county council is reimbursed for the rest from the National Social Insurance. The Seven Crown Reform also directly affected the patient's choice of doctors and doctors' salary levels, as will be detailed later.

4. *Maternity and Child Benefits.* These include complete coverage of prenatal care, delivery by midwives in a hospital, infant care at child-welfare centers, cash grants of $180/yr for each child, and school medical care for children.

The outstanding feature of the Swedish Social Insurance scheme is that all Swedes have equal coverage and, hence, equal access to all types of medical care, independent of their salary level, social status, or health condition. On the other hand, complete insurance coverage, which is compulsory, is accompanied by high taxes and loss of individual choice in selecting health coverage plans.

Cost

Sweden's expenditures for social welfare and health care comprise a large percentage of the total government outlay. For 1970 to 1971, social welfare expenses, including health care, were 28 percent of the total government expenses compared to 17 percent for education and only 13 percent for military expenses. Health costs in 1969 were 1.4 billion dollars, which represented 5:5 percent of Sweden's gross national product. These costs are increasing at a rate of about 7 percent/yr. In 1971, the Swedish county councils spent 78 percent of their total budget or 2 billion dollars (about $250 per person) on medical care. This represented an eightfold increase compared to expenses in 1960.

The system for health and social welfare is tax-financed and because health and social benefits are so comprehensive total tax rates are high. For example, a married man earning $4,000 a year pays 41 percent of his salary for total taxes, while a man earning $10,000 a year pays 60 percent.

Levels of Medical Care

The first priority of Swedish medical care planners has been to establish its excellent system of regional hospitals. However, medical care starts when the patient is first sick or injured, i.e., when he seeks primary (or first contact) medical care. If his illness is severe or he needs evaluation by a specialist, he is referred to an intermediate specialist-care facility which is either the central polyclinics or the hospital outpatient clinics. If more extensive diagnostic evaluation is needed, medical treatment, or surgery, he is admitted to a hospital, usually first to a district hospital. If more specialized diagnosis or treatment is required than the district hospital can provide, he is transferred to a larger central hospital or to one of seven regional hospitals.

Primary Medical Care

There has been a dramatic increase in demand for primary medical care so that growing importance is being placed on the care of outpatients to relieve the pressures for hospitalization. There was an increase in ambulatory visits to doctors of 250 percent, from 7.4 to 18.7 million visits annually from 1952 to 1966.

Whereas hospital care in Sweden is almost all under government auspices, primary medical care is provided by both government physicians and a dwindling supply of private physicians. The government provides general practitioners or district medical officers (DMO). It also runs the ambulance service and provides district nurses, district midwives, maternity centers and child welfare centers (often adjacent to hospitals), a school health service, tuberculosis centers, and a public dental service. Private physicians practice in offices and rarely have access to hospital practices; they practice either alone or in multispecialty doctors' groups (Läkarhus). Private physicians also staff the night emergency service (Larmtjänst). Other areas of private medicine are in industry and in preventive medicine centers.

District Medical Officer. There are about 800 DMOs in Sweden and they account for more than 23 percent of all outpatient visits. In the sparsely populated rural areas where the DMO is the only physician available, he often is responsible for maternity and child welfare, school health, nursing homes, and public health work as well. Although the national goal is one DMO per 4,000 people, the DMO in the rural areas serves a population of about 6,000 people. In cities such as Göteborg, a DMO's district encompasses 10,000 to 25,000 persons.

The DMO for Västra Frölunda, a planned "satellite town," describes his day: from 8:00 A.M. to 1:00 P.M. he is scheduled to see 25 to 35 patients from his district; from 1:00 P.M. to 5:00 P.M. he holds private office hours in the same office, during which time he sees 10 to 15 patients, some of whom choose to come to him from outside his district. Thus, he sees 35 to 50 patients a day or about six patients an hour. He works five days a week and is on call at night.

The district patients pay a fee of seven crowns ($1.40) and social insurance reimburses the Göteborg county council, which operates the clinic, $4.05 for each patient. Thus, for each outpatient visit the county council collects $5.45 with which it pays for the expenses of the DMO's office and pays his salary. In Göteborg, "mixed DMOs," who see both public and private patients, are allowed to supplement their salary with private practice fees and they make excellent salaries compared to hospital physicians who receive salaries only. However, this is not representative of most other parts of Sweden, since almost all DMOs elsewhere work on a fixed-salary fixed-time basis. There are plans to eliminate the remaining "mixed DMOs" and put all DMOs on a strict salary basis seeing public patients full time.

The DMO's patients are not unlike those of his counterpart, the American general practitioner. Since his district has many young families, he sees many children. Mostly he deals with minor illnesses and treats more than 90 percent of his patients himself. He has only five to ten minutes per patient and too many patients with minor illnesses occupy time that would be better spent with the more seriously ill.

The DMO whom I visited thinks it is wise for all doctors to have general practice experience. However, like most young physicians in Sweden, his eventual aim is for a career in hospital practice and research. The hospital-based specialty training that most young doctors now receive makes full-time careers in primary patient-care seem unattractive, but the need for such physicians exists both in the country and in the city.

Solo Private Practice. Of the approximately 10,000 physicians in Sweden, an estimated 1,350 or 14 percent are in private practice. Of these, about 400 are over age sixty-five and work only part time. The total number of physicians in private practice decreases yearly as the older physicians retire and only a few young ones take their place. Of the 1,200 general practitioners in Sweden, 400 are in private practice, while 800 are government-employed DMOs. Other private physicians function as specialists, such as otolaryngologists and clinical cardiologists. Private physicians provide 26 percent of the care for ambulatory patients.

Since no private physicians have staff privileges at government hospitals, the practice of most of them is limited to their own offices. For this reason, almost no surgeons are in private practice since they would not have access to a hospital where they could operate. If a patient requires hospitalization, he will almost certainly be admitted to a government hospital where his private physician can no longer care for him. Thus, the mutual advantage of a well-developed doctor-patient relationship is lost. For the physician, exclusion from hospital care means loss of access to advanced diagnostic facilities and absence of stimulation from colleagues, consultants, and teaching sessions, thus dissuading young Swedish physicians from entering private practice. Instead, they prefer to stay on the hospital staff, often remaining in a junior position for many years. During 1970 in Göteborg, which has 196 private practitioners, many of them past retirement age, *not one* young physician entered private pratice as noted by N. S. Blume, MD (written communication, August 1971).

According to Nils Blume, MD, former president of the Göteborg Medical Society, young doctors are dissuaded from entering private practice both by the counterattractions of modern hospital-based medicine and by Sweden's prevailing viewpoint that it is not right to earn money from ill people, at least not in private practice. While the future of Swedish private practice is uncertain because of the government's stated goal of total socialization, Dr. Blume sees some signs of respite, namely, the rising costs of medical care and the increased output of new physicians during poor financial times, making the government unwilling to assume all the costs of Sweden's medical care. Also, some of the public still insist on a visit to a private physician as an alternative to long waits and long lines at government hospitals.

Private Group Practice. In order to attract more young physicians into nongovernmental medical practice, the Swedish Medical Society in 1963 started to construct "doctors' houses" (Läkarhus) to provide office space and diagnostic facilities for new multispecialty group practices. About 260 physicians are now employed by the Swedish Doctors Service Corporation (Läkartjänst AB), which has organized private group practices in four cities.

The aim of these doctors' houses was to permit young physicians to have modern facilities to treat outpatients outside of the hospital setting and to allow the patient total medical care. The corporation supplies managerial personnel to handle the business side of the practice. Each doctor's net earnings, after expenses, are directly proportional to his income from patient fees and reimbursement from national insurance. Incomes equal or exceed government salaries for doctors.

Physicians like the practice of medicine in the doctors' houses. For example, the radiologist for the Göteborg group enjoys foremost the freedom to make professional decisions that he did not have when working in large government hospitals. For patients, "doctors' house" provides more personalized medical service than the government hospital outpatient clinic. Whether or not the doctor's house will continue to operate on a private basis is still uncertain.

Emergency Care. The Director of the Emergency Medical Service (Larmtjänst) in Göteborg, Björn Lindholm, MD, explained that two physicians with radios in their cars cover the entire city of Göteborg every night and weekend and make emergency house calls.

Each physician on call sees 10 to 15 patients a night. The Larmtjänst doctors do not respond to every call themselves. All calls are screened by trained operators. The waiting period between the call and the doctor's arrival at the house varies between thirty minutes and five hours. The operators assign the most serious cases first. The cost to a patient for a house call is $3; the doctor is reimbursed an additional $14 from the government for each call.

The primary usefulness of Larmtjänst is that it fills an immense vacuum in the Swedish medical care system, that is, no other provision is made by the government for delivering home care to patients during nights and weekends. Both the district medical offices and the hospital outpatient clinics are closed at night. Thus, a patient without his "own doctor" (most Swedish patients) has two choices if he is sick at night: go to a hospital emergency room, which might mean a four-hour to six-hour wait before he is seen, or call the Larmtjänst.

The emergency medical service or Larmtjänst, although limited to the physician's black bag and marked by a lack of continuity of treatment, provides prompt home medical evaluations for those who cannot come to the hospital at night.

Ambulance Service. One excellent aspect of emergency medical services in Göteborg is a well-staffed city ambulance service equipped with twenty-five modern ambulances assigned by a central dispatcher. The ambulance attendants are city firemen who have received a minimum of three months of hospital training, two months of which are spent in the operating room assisting an anesthetist and learning resuscitation techniques by first-hand experience.

Industrial Medicine. One other important area of non-governmental primary medical care in Sweden is in the field of industrial medicine. The largest companies operate and finance their own clinics near their factories.

Intermediate (Specialist) Care

District Central Polyclinic. When a specialist is needed, the DMO can refer the patient to district central polyclinics. In Västra Frölunda, for example, the central polyclinic has doctors in eleven different specialties. Operating rooms are available for minor surgery. Public health nurses and midwives are responsible for prenatal and postnatal "mother's care" and for a comprehensive program of infant care.

Hospital Emergency Room. The hospital emergency room evaluates patients who come in on their own or by ambulance and patients referred by primary doctors. Göteborg, with only one large general hospital, the Sahlgrenska, is unique because almost all emergencies in this city are sent to this one facility.

Only about 10 percent of the patients seen are admitted to the hospital. Unless a patient obviously needs immediate admission or can be sent home, he is kept in the overnight ward for further observation which may decide whether hospital admission is essential.

The chief of the emergency room and the many patients I talked to are dissatisfied with the current quarters. The rooms are few and cramped and staffing is sparse. It requires heroic Scandinavian patience to be a patient—or a physician —in Sweden.

Hospital Outpatient Clinics. An estimated 50 percent of the 18.4 million ambulatory-patient visits in 1966 took place in hospital outpatient departments, which are becoming increasingly busy each year.

Before the Seven Crown Reform in January 1970, both hospital service chiefs and junior staff physicians had been permitted to see private patients on a fee-for-service basis in the clinics run by each of the hospital's services, as well as to see "service patients." Since the Seven Crown Reform, no physicians are permitted to see private patients in the clinics and all hospital physicians are on salary.

All patients I talked to complained about the long waiting time for an appointment, which ranges from three weeks for a "semiemergency" to six months for a nonemergency. Patients dislike not being able to request the doctor of their choice and usually having to see a different doctor each visit.

The good result of the reform for patients was on the

financial side. Now they pay only seven crowns ($1.40) per visit, which covers doctors' services, X-ray films, and laboratory costs.

Most of the staff physicians in the medical clinics told me they were not happy with the effects of the Seven Crown Reform. Several admitted frankly that the total shift from private patients to randomly assigned "service patients" whom they see only for one visit caused them to take much less of a personal interest in each patient. The doctors admitted that they spent less time with the patient, scheduled his return appointment at longer intervals, and referred patients more readily to other clinics. According to Lars Werkö, MD, Chief of Medicine in Göteborg, "many hospital-based physicians regard their work now with an apathy previously unknown."

Maternity Care. Prospective mothers have monthly appointments at the Obstetrics Clinic without charge. However, this requires several hours of waiting in the clinic and the mother sees a different obstetrician at each visit unless she is willing to pay an $8 fee each time for scheduling her visits with the same obstetrician. This physician will not, however, deliver her baby. If the delivery is uncomplicated, it will be performed in the hospital by a nurse-midwife whom the mother has not met. If complications are expected, an obstetrician is called. On the other hand, if some mothers miss the luxury of a "personal obstetrician," no one objects to the results that Swedish maternal care produces—lowest infant mortality in the world.

Hospitals

. . . The patient is admitted to a four-bed room since no private or semiprivate rooms are available. All expenses of hospitalization, including room, food, physician's salary, X-ray film and laboratory expenses, and drugs, will be paid by the county council, which operates the hospital.

The patient never has his choice of doctor, but is assigned the doctor in his ward who is often a specialist. The hospital doctors are full-time salaried government employees; many in the regional hospitals also hold university teaching appointments.

One big difference in the ward routine from an American hospital is that the nursing staff is given more responsibility. The nurse can alter the treatments the doctor suggests on rounds on her own initiative and in an emergency or when the doctor is not available if the patient's needs change.

Comment

Although Sweden's bed-to-population ratio is the highest in the world, in practice there are long waiting lists of patients to be admitted to hospitals. A patient may have to wait a year for elective surgery. This is because many wards are not open to patients due to staff shortages (6.4 percent of positions for physicians and 5.8 percent of nursing positions went unfilled in 1971). Sweden hopes to correct these shortages by enrollment of more medical and nursing students. Also, open elective beds are often in short supply because many are filled by relatively well patients who would be treated on an ambulatory basis in the United States. However, acute cases are always admitted for care.

One of the most cutting criticism of Swedish medical care is the charge that a Swedish patient "has many doctors but no doctor," since a different physician will probably treat him for each hospitalization and each outpatient visit to the hospital. The patient is often shunted between different specialty wards and clinics for brief consultations with different specialists. The "personal physician" is rapidly becoming extinct in Sweden. The few, mostly older, physicians who do carry out this function are prohibited from caring for their patients in the hospital but must defer to the full-time hospital specialist. Therefore, the advantages of a close doctor-patient relationship do not carry into the hospital setting when a new physician takes over the case. The relationship between a hospital patient and a Swedish hospital specialist is traditionally a formal one. The physician is well versed in the patient's medical problem but seldom knows much about him as a person.

But again the disadvantage of the loss of a "personal physician" must be balanced with the advantages of a system that provides well-trained physicians available to diagnose and treat all citizens for any serious illness, an advantage not all Americans can claim. An ideal system would combine the personal knowledge and concern of an American "personal physician" with equal access to specialists and to efficient medical facilities which are the right and usually the reality of every Swede.

Starting in January 1973, the nominal fee that the patient himself pays for medical services in Sweden has been increased from 7 crowns to 12 crowns (approximately $2.75) for each outpatient visit. For drugs, the patient will pay a maximum of $3.00 for any prescription or group of prescriptions on the same day. National health insurance supports ambulatory-patient care by paying fees to the county for each outpatient visit, which have been increased from $6.00 to $14.75 since January 1 [1973]. Also, it supports hospital care by $2.00/day/patient. The patients pay nothing for their hospitalization, but receive compensation proportional to their incomes while in the hospital. Hospitals are owned, operated, and financed almost totally by the county councils. Present hospital expenses in Sweden are $80 to $100/patient/day in the central hospitals, which include physicians' salaries. Preventive health-care services (except for children and expectant mothers) and dental services are not covered by national health insurance.

BIBLIOGRAPHY

An asterisk (*) preceding a reference indicates that the article or part of it has been reprinted in this book.

BOOKS

Alford, R. R. Health care politics: ideological and interest-group barriers to reform. University of Chicago Press. '75.

Bloch, L. W. and others. Analyzing health care policy; a resource guide. (Pamphlet No. 255) Joint Council on Economic Education. 1212 Avenue of the Americas. New York, NY 10036. '77.

Crichton, Michael. Five patients: the hospital explained. Knopf. '70.

Duffy, John. The healers: the rise of the medical establishment. McGraw-Hill. '76.

Ehrenreich, Barbara and Ehrenreich, John. The American health empire: power, profits, and politics. Random House. '70.

Fuchs, V. R. Essays in the economics of health and medical care. National Bureau of Economic Research, Inc. 261 Madison Ave. New York, NY 10016. '72.

Fuchs, V. R. Who shall live? health economics, and social choice. Basic Books. '74.

Grossman, H. R. For health's sake; a critical analysis of medical care in the United States. Pacific Books. '77.

Haag, J. H. Consumer health: products and services. Lea & Febiger. '75.

Illich, I. D. Medical nemesis; the expropriation of health. Pantheon. '76.

Kennedy, E. M. In critical condition: the crisis in America's health care. Simon & Schuster. '72.

Klaw, Spencer. The great American medicine show: the unhealthy state of U.S. medical care, and what can be done about it. Viking. '75.

Schwartz, Harry. The case for American medicine: a realistic look at our health care system. McKay. '72.

PERIODICALS

Aging. 274:32 Ag. '77. Survey shows Medicaid money is misspent.

American Heritage. 28:96-105. Je. '77. Belly-my-grizzle; herbal medicine. Spencer Klaw.

*Blair & Ketchum's Country Journal. 3:71-7. Ap. '76. The rural health care crisis. J. B. Dunne.

Bulletin of the Atomic Scientists. 33:38-43. S. '77. Rx: a peer review system for physicians. Jacob Fine.

*Business Week. p 74-6. My. 30, '77. Containing the cost of employee health plans: health maintenance organizations.

Business Week. p 38-9. Ag. 15, '77. Unhealthy state of coalfield health care; 50 clinics.

Changing Times: 30:15-17. Mr. '76. What's going on in health care.

Changing Times. 30:13-16. Jl. '76. Costs of having a baby today.

Commonweal. 104:451-2. Jl. 22, '77. New abortion debate; Supreme Court decision on Medicaid funding.

Consumer Reports. 41:185-6. Ap. '76. Health insurance for older people: filling the gaps in Medicare [discussion].

Consumer Reports. 42:544-8, 598-601. S., O. '77. Medical malpractice.

Current. 180:48-50. F. '76. Don't give physicians too much power [interview]. E. D. Pellegrino.

*Current History. 72:193-5+. My./Je. '77. Health care in America: an overview; symposium.
  Reprinted in this volume: Federal involvement in health care after 1945. L. R. Judd. p 200-6+; Health employment and the nation's health. C. E. Bishop. p 208-9; Health facilities in the United States. D. P. Rice. p 211-12.

*Current History. 73:1-31+. Jl./Ag. '77. Improving health care in America; symposium.
  Reprinted in this volume: Health care and the patient's needs. M. W. Herman. p 1-4+; The right to health care. B. B. Page. p 5-8+; The British national health service in international perspective. J. G. Simanis. p 27-9+.

Daedalus. 106:1-278. Winter '77. Doing better and feeling worse: health in the United States.

*Dun's Review. 109:23+. My. '77. Kaiser and the "desert doctors"; a way to cut medical bills. Lee Smith.

Dun's Review. 109:48-53+. My. '77. Race to cut medical costs. Arlene Hershman.

Dun's Review. 110:105-6+. N. '77. Growth power in hospital-supply stocks; interview, ed. by Arlene Hershman. Frederick Prunier.

Editorial Research Reports. v 2, no 5:603-20. Ag. 9, '74. Health maintenance organizations. Mary Costello.

*Environment. 18:6-18. My. '76. American medicine. R. B. Greifinger and V. W. Sidel.

Family Health. 8:29-31+. Jl. '76. Why doctors don't make house calls; interviews ed. by J. R. Kesselman and Franklynn Peterson.

Family Health. 9:36-9+. Ap. '77. Country doctor; work of Garrett Duckworth in Mound City, Kan. Charles Remsberg.

Forbes. 119:53-4. My. 15, '77. Carter's stab at health care.

Forbes. 119:67-8. Je. 1, '77. Medical technology: too much of a good thing?

Forbes. 120:40-6. O. 1, '77. Physician, heal thyself . . . or else!

House & Garden. 148:94-5+. S. '76. Is American medicine killing us? views of Ivan D. Illich; with comments by physicians. John Wykert.

Intellect. 105:168-70. D. '76. Preventive medicine may be hazardous to your pocketbook. S. O. Schweitzer.

Intellect. 106:100-1. S. '77. Governmental interference with medical care; excerpts from addresses. D. X. Freedman.

Intellect. 106:149-51. O. '77. Paraprofessionals in a multiservice community mental health center. M. B. Ahmed and Arnold Birenbaum.

*JAMA (Journal of the American Medical Association). 223:1369-75. Mr. 19, '73. Medical care in Sweden; lessons for America. J. L. Andrews Jr.

McCall's. 105:169+. N. '77. Is your doctor overcharging you? W. A. Nolen.

Monthly Labor Review. 100:50. My. '77. Supply of federal physicians and dentists found adequate.

Nation. 222:785-8. Je. 26, '76. Clinics, toilets, & black management: health care in the rural South; Beaufort-Jasper comprehensive health services. Scott Graber and Susan Graber.

Nation. 224:242-4. F. 26, '77. Model for fraud: Michigan's Medicaid rip-off. E. E. Chen.

Nation. 225:210-12. S. 10, '77. Medical inflation: the system is the sickness. G. A. Silver.

*National Observer. p 5. Ja. 17, '76. Medicaid retrenchment. R. W. Merry.

*National Observer. p 6. O. 30, '76. Your doctor is cramming. Patrick Young.

*National Observer. p 2. Mr. 26, '77. The "rich" Medicare docs: misleading figures. Lawrence Mosher.

*National Observer. p 12. Ap. 23, '77. AMA president discusses health-care costs; interview with Dr. Richard Palmer. Sheila McGough.

*National Review. 25:780-4+. Jl. 20, '73. The high cost of health. Alan Reynolds.
    Discussion: National Review. 25:920+, 972, 1153+. Ag. 31, S. 14, O. 26, '73.

National Review. 29:1368. N. 25, '77. Uncle Sam's dangerous prescriptions. M. Stanton Evans.

Nation's Business. 65:16-20. F. '77. How business can help cut health-care costs.

New Republic. 176:22-3. Mr. 12; 16-19 Mr. 19; 11-15 Ap. 16; 22-5 My. 28; 177:9-2, Jl. 2, '77. Anatomy of health care costs. Eliot Marshall.

New Republic. 177:11. S. 3, '77. Pushy parents; question of law requiring medical schools to admit American transfers from abroad. K. Keegan.

*New York Times. sec IV, p 11. F. 1, '76. U.S. doctors: about 5 percent are unfit.

*New York Times. p 23. Ap. 27, '77. Well, who needs life savings? J. P. Allegrante.

New York Times. p 22. D. 19, '77. U.S. planners see little hope of obtaining national health insurance.

New York Times Magazine. p 108-9+. Jl. 4, '76. Dark secret of doctors: most things get better by themselves; interview, ed. by Lee Edson. Lewis Thomas.

*New York Times Magazine. p 12-13+. Ja. 9, '77. National health insurance—the dream whose time has come? R. J. Margolis.

*Newsweek. 89:4. Ja. 10, '77. Why people are mad at doctors. Maurice Fox.

Newsweek. 89:64-5. F. 28, '77. Treating the old and the sick. M. Clark and M. Gosnell.

Newsweek. 89:96. Mr. 7, '77. Hot seat: Joseph Califano of HEW. G. F. Will.

*Newsweek. 89:84+. My. 9, '77. Health-cost crisis. Matt Clark and others.

Newsweek. 90:60+. O. 10, '77. Medicine: a decade behind; U.S.-Soviet comparison. Matt Clark and others.

Newsweek. 90:105+. N. 21, '77. It's an emergency! Peter Bonventre and others.

Progressive. 41:9-10. Ja. '77. Our ailing health system.

Progressive. 41:16-19. O. '77. Health care: the problem is profits. Bernard Winter.

*Public Interest. 48:40-54. Summer '77. The high cost of hospitals —and what to do about it. Martin Feldstein.

Reader's Digest. 111:122-6. O. '77. What's wrong with U.S. health care? J. A. Califano Jr.

Saturday Review. 5:10-13+. Ja. 7, '78. The great health care rip-off. Robert Claiborne.

Science. 192:105-11. Ap. 9, '76. Scientific basis for the support of biomedical science. J. H. Comroe Jr. and R. D. Dripps.

Science. 194:700-4. N. 12. '76. Health manpower act: aid but not comfort for medical schools. B. J. Culliton.

Science. 194:1013-20. D. 3, '76. Life events, stress, and illness. J. G. Rabkin and E. L. Struening.

Science. 195:457-62. F. 4, '77. Health economics and preventive care. M. M. Kristein and others.

Science. 196:129-36. Ap. 8, '77. Need for a new medical model: a challenge for biomedicine. G. L. Engel.

Science. 197:1062-3. S. 9, '77. Future doctors balk at the [medical school] bill. L. J. Carter.

Science. 197:1066. S. 9, '77. Four medical schools draw the line on capitation. B. J. Culliton.

Science Digest. 79:42-5. F. '76. Everything is bad for your health. Frank Kendig.

Science Digest. 80:78-80. Jl. '76. Big government's medical headache. D. S. Greenberg.

Science Digest. 81:62-4. My. '77. New breed of doctor: he'll know you better.

Science Digest. 81:8-11+. Je. '77. Impaired MDs now recognized as a peril to patients. Marvin Grosswirth.

*Scientific American. 229:22-52+. S. '73. Life and death and medicine; symposium.
   Bibliography. p 198+.
   Reprinted in this volume: The medical business. J. L. Goddard. p 161-6.

Senior Scholastic. 109:22-3. O. 21, '76. Health care: can the U.S. learn from other countries?

Senior Scholastic. 109:2-4+. Ap. 21, '77. Health care, U.S.A.

Society. 14:41-6. Ja. '77. Emergency medicine. Harry Perlstadt and L. J. Kozak.

Time. 108:60-2. Ag. 9, '76. Struggle to stay healthy. J. H. Knowles.

*Time. 109:73. Ja. 17, '77. How nurses rate hospital care.

Time. 110:94. O. 3, '77. Federal money talks; transfer of students from foreign schools.

U.S. News & World Report. 80:18-20. Mr. 22, '76. Billions in Medicaid ripoffs; can anyone stop it?

U.S. News & World Report. 80:36-8. Mr. 29, '76. What hospitals are doing to cut down accidents.

U.S. News & World Report. 82:35-40+. Mr. 28, '77. Uproar over medical bills; with interview with W. J. McNerney. J. Mann.

U.S. News & World Report. 82:62. Ap. 4, '77. Prevention or cure? Behind the shift in health care. A. T. Brett.

*U.S. News & World Report. 82:43-5. My. 23, '77. New medical technology: is it worth the price? A. T. Brett.

U.S. News & World Report. 83:50-2+. O. 17, '77. America's doctors: a profession in trouble. A. T. Brett.

Vital Speeches of the Day. 43:211-15. Ja. 15, '77. Business looks at health care costs; address, November 18, 1976. J. H. Perkins.

Vital Speeches of the Day. 43:700-2. S. 1, '77. Rationed care; address, June 19, 1977. R. E. Palmer.

Vital Speeches of the Day. 43:753-6. O. 1, '77. Health costs containment; address, August 9, 1977. W. E. Ryan.

Vital Speeches of the Day. 44:19-21. O. 15, '77. Health of our children; proposed Child Health Assessment Act; address, September 9, 1977. J. A. Califano.

*Washington Post. p C 1. Mr. 7, '76. Rx for health care—a national authority. C. C. Edwards.

*Washington Post. p A 8. S. 7, '76. N.Y. doctors fight "Medicaid mill" tag. D. C. Berliner.

*Working Papers for a New Society. 4:18-19+. Winter '77. A coming doctor surplus? Paul Starr.